I0428687

ISBN: 1463575548

ISBN-13: 978-1463575540

Printed in USA by Marashlian, Inc.

F I T   L E A N   &   H E A L T H Y

8 Simple Steps

Table of Contents

"The only good is knowledge and the only evil is ignorance." Socrates

INTRODUCTION

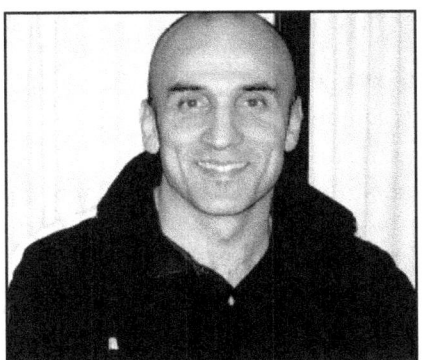

As a professional trainer for more than 25 years I get a lot of fitness information coming in my direction on a daily basis. This information comes from as many sources as you can dream of, some scientific, some not; some factual and a lot of fiction. Part of being a professional is to be able to sift through the junk, the half-truths, falsehoods or exaggerated information to find the key pearls or senior truths that work on the majority of people each time over when applied correctly.

Not All Information Is of Equal Importance

I have observed 3 basic types of information that one should be aware of:

Vital information (the Gems). These are the key senior fundamental facts. The most important, useful and valuable facts.

Usable information (the Good). These are useful and valuable but not as important as the vital information. Not all facts are equal.

Completely false and useless information (the Ugly). This is the stuff you really need to avoid. This useless information will waste your time and can hurt or harm you.

Learn From Credible, Experienced and Proven Sources

Whose advice do you take? The celebrity, the doctor, the expert internet marketer, the twenty-two year-old trainer, the jock, the "know-it-all", Mama, Papa, the scientist, the businessman or Mr. Money Bags?

Having some idea and being able to recognize the similarities and differences between the three basic types of information can save you a lot of time, money and heart-ache. Being able to recognize false, misleading or misrepresented data given by corrupt experts with vested interests and pseudo experts is vital to anyone's success.

Here are some quick tips to help you discern the difference between the Gems, the Good and Ugly types of information:

Who wrote it or who is saying it?

Does he/she have any formal education in the area?

Is he/she an expert in the field being communicated about?

Does he/she have a proven track record and results in the field? If so, can these be verified?

Does he/she have any vested or monetary interest in the product being communicated about?

RELIABLE SOURCES: Are mostly those who do not have a vested interest and are not employed by someone with a vested interest in promoting lies or bad products. Some examples of Reliable Sources in the health and fitness fields may be: exercise scientists, physiologists, kinesiologists, research institutes and some professional trainers. Their information might be relayed through books, magazines, journals, DVDs, videos, seminars, one-on-one coaching, personal training or the internet.

UNRELIABLE SOURCES: There is no real limit to where these unreliable sources come from. Some of the more common ones are: well-intentioned but mis-informed friends, relatives and associates; not so well-intentioned experts/professionals with vested interests.

VERY UNRELIABLE AND UNTRUSTWORTHY SOURCES: These are individuals or groups with vested interests. Their interest is purely financial and they can come from many different areas. The most common ones are some internet marketers - those people who find a "niche" and promote products with little knowledge or care of the true results. These people flock to health and fitness because just about anyone with a body is interested in improving their health and fitness - it's a huge market packed with less than valuable information and products.

At the end of the day what really counts or matters and the only test worth considering is whether or not information or a fact works. Period!

I have put together some vital information (Gems) so you can safely and intelligently navigate your way to a healthier, fitter, stronger and more toned you. This is an action book; my goal is to get you achieving your fitness and wellness goals right away. So be prepared and may your life never be the same again.

Rudi Marashlian
Exercise Science, Applied Science

HOW TO USE THIS BOOK

Here is an eight-step program that will successfully walk you through the confusing maze of contradictory information that exists on exercise and diets so that you can truly get the body you want. It is intended that you will use this book as a workbook and that it will get written on and maybe even dog-eared in a few places.

Just start at the beginning, Step One, and continue through the book doing each step, one at a time and in order. The most logical place to start is with your goals and once you do "Step One - Name Your Goals", the book will help guide you in selecting the right activities to achieve those goals. From there you will be taken through a few more vital steps including a simple diet review and tips to propel you in the right direction so that achieving your goals can become a reality.

My purpose in writing this book is to get you started with exercising and doing the right activities to achieve your personal fitness goals. It may be that you only get through the first few steps in this book and find yourself enthusiastically working out, feeling great and getting results. That's fine. Go for it, but if you reach a point where you need a bit more guidance then go back and work through more of this book. What I'm trying to say here is, this book is yours to use however it works best for you. You can go through the whole book step by step or get started as soon as you feel confident and ready. The choice is yours.

This book mirrors the format I use with my clients to get them up and started towards success. The idea is to reproduce the great results my clients get with one-on-one training in a book format so many people can have access to this workable system. One person at a time, while workable, is the slow way to help many people get into great shape and experience the fantastic health benefits of correct exercise and diet.

Here's to a future of health, strength and fitness for you.

CLIENT TESTIMONIALS

"I have hit every goal so far on time. I've added 6 pounds of lean muscle, lost 4 pounds of fat and 2 inches off my abdomen in just 7 weeks. My energy level has gone through the roof and my strength has become powerful.

"Rudi is by far the highest quality trainer I've ever met."

Armen, Venture Capitalist
Age 31

"I have trained with Rudi for two years now and have noticed a wonderful improvement in my strength and cardio. I feel much lighter (I have lost inches for sure) and yet very strong.

"I am 52 years old but I do not look or feel my age.

"Most important is how this body feels. As you get older, working long days, kids, whatever you have to handle, it's easy to feel like a tired slouchy donut by the end of the day. When you are fit you really hang better. Your energy is better. There's an "aliveness" there when you push the body and keep it fit.

Debbie, Business Owner
Age 52

"My body has obviously changed as I've dropped 2 sizes in the last 6 months. Previously I hid my arms with sleeves or sweaters to cover the "bat" arms, but those days are over! I proudly wear tank tops or go sleeveless with confidence and let the arms glow. I was recently asked by a complete stranger where I train, validation my body is responding nicely.

"My workouts are amazing, Rudi tailors every training session to MY needs and goals. I continue to learn new techniques and tools, and feel with 100% certainty I could never have made my progress to date without you, Rudi. Thank you!"

Sherryl, Business Executive
Age 57

"I was a physical mess. My body was so out of shape that I could not bend down or put my socks on without getting out of breath. My thought was that I was in no shape to work out so I felt hopeless in my goal of being in shape. Working with Rudi put the hope back. I can run, jump, bend, and yes, put my socks on without feeling like I'm about to take my last breath."

Ray, Photographer
Age 39

"Rudi's emphasis on correct form during every exercise and slow versus fast movements, helped me to build muscles without injury. He showed me how to use machines or my own body weight to exercise.

"Now I can lift the 52-pound bag of dog food off the warehouse store shelf - something I could not do before. I can balance on one leg to tie my shoe, without leaning or holding onto something like I did before. My posture has improved and I've learned how to work out safely."

Linda, Real Estate Agent
Age 61

"I am just 3 months into working with Rudi twice a week. I am starting to see a great deal of improvement in my fitness and strength. I recently competed in an off-road motorcycle race, The Silver State 300, and I could see a huge improvement in my fitness. After finishing a 65 mile leg of the race I easily felt like I could have done another leg with no problem. Three months ago it would have been impossible to have raced at this level without being exhausted!"

David, Business Executive
Age 52

"I am pushing myself (my body) more and I'm winning more than the body is. It's pushing back and resisting but I'm more successful at making it do what I want anyway."

Sandee, Business Executive
Age 56

"Nothing happens unless we first dream." Carl Sandburg

"The invariable mark of a dream is to see it come true." Ralph Waldo-Emerson

STEP ONE - NAME YOUR GOALS

STEP ONE - NAME YOUR GOALS

TOP FOUR FITNESS GOALS

1. Weight loss, lose fat, trim down to look good

2. Build muscle, firm and tone to look good

3. Improve health, energy and vitality to feel good

4. Rehabilitation, fix an injury to improve function

SIX FITNESS TOOLS

The unlimited benefits of being physically fit are well known and documented. Below are six of the most basic types of fitness tools that people are interested in:

BODY COMPOSITION: *the ratio or amount of lean (muscle) to fat tissue (affects health and appearance).* There is hardly a person on Planet Earth who doesn't have some interest in either losing body fat or increasing lean tissue or both. This will involve diet, strength and cardio training.

DIET AND NUTRITION: *the ratio or amount of protein, fats and carbohydrates, water, vitamins and minerals will have quite an impact on your results.*

STRENGTH: *muscle strength and tone (affects function, quality of life and appearance).* The more conditioned muscles are, the more calories you will burn. The stronger you become, the easier daily activities become and the less likely it will be to injure your back, knees and other vital areas of the body.

AEROBIC/CARDIO: *heart and lung improvements (affects heart and lung health and helps you to feel good).* The more heart and lung fitness you have the easier endurance activities become. Cardio-vascular fitness helps give you a feeling of energy and strengthens the heart, lungs, circulatory system and more. Aerobic exercise/fitness also helps burn calories.

FLEXIBILITY: *improves range of joint movements (for function and quality of movement and helps relieve those tight spots).* The more flexible your joints and muscles, the easier your daily activities become and the less likely you are to injure your back, knees, shoulders and other areas of the body.

REHABILITATION: *fixing weak links or injured body areas (for function, stability and quality of life).*

STEP ONE - NAME YOUR GOALS

When a sedentary person starts to exercise weak links will commonly appear. This is useful as you can then repair the weak link. It is better for the link to appear under a controlled environment instead of giving out during an emergency when you need the body, body part or area to function at maximal effort or 100% without failing you.

The above five basic areas of fitness should help you in naming your fitness goals. These are all measurable and will help you track your progress and results.

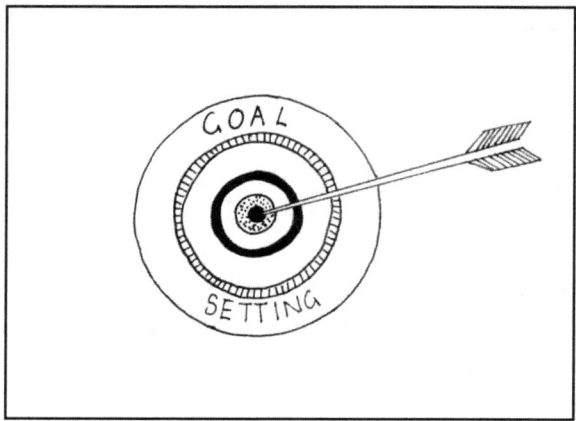

Before you set off on any journey you will need to have some idea of where you want to end up otherwise you will have no idea of which way to go and could more than likely end up going around in circles.

Every trip has a starting place, a route and a final destination. Every activity in life should have goals to achieve. A logical place to start in order to achieve any goal is to precisely name what it is you really want to achieve. If you never clearly name or delineate what it is you want to achieve, how will you be able to make a plan to get there or know when you are there?

Goals set the direction of all planning and actions and help keep you motivated along the way.

A good first step in starting towards attaining any goal is to write it down clearly, so go to the next page and let's get started!

STEP ONE - NAME YOUR GOALS

1. WHAT DO YOU WANT TO ACHIEVE THAT WOULD MAKE YOU REALLY HAPPY?

Clearly define your top three health or fitness goals and write them below.

Goal 1:	
Goal 2:	
Goal 3:	

2. WHAT REALISTIC TIME FRAME DO YOU WISH TO ACHIEVE YOUR GOALS?

Circle a time frame from the choices below.

1-3 months 3-6 months 6-9 months 9-12 months other: _____

3. WHAT IS YOUR LEVEL OF INTEREST AND COMMITMENT TO ACHIEVING YOUR GOALS?

Circle the appropriate level to indicate your level of commitment to achieving your goals.

50% 60% 70% 80% 90% 100%

4. WHAT IS YOUR LEVEL OF WILLINGNESS TO DO WHATEVER IT TAKES TO SUCCEED?

Circle the appropriate level to indicate level of willingness.

50% 60% 70% 80% 90% 100%

The degree of success and failure in achieving your goals has a lot to do with your level of interest, commitment and action. Let's just do it!

Now go to Step 2 where you will work out which physical activities you should be doing to achieve the goals you wrote in the chart above.

"Lack of activity destroys the good condition of every human being while movement and methodical physical exercise save and preserve it." Plato

STEP TWO - MATCH YOUR ACTIONS TO YOUR GOALS

STEP TWO - MATCH YOUR ACTIONS TO YOUR GOALS

Now that you've decided on the top three goals for your body it's time to work out exactly what activities you'll need to do in order to best achieve them. Not all activities achieve the same results and it's very important to know what activities match with your specific goals.

EXERCISE FOR PURPOSE NOT JUST ENJOYMENT

Choose exercises or workouts based on your GOALS. It's also good to choose activities you like but more importantly, they also have to be able to achieve your goals. Priority one goes to activities that match and achieve your goals.

For example, Marsha loves to walk but her goal is to get a stronger and more toned body. Walking does not do that, so she will also need to include strength exercises to achieve her goals.

Peter has a really tight back and finds it difficult to bend down to pick up things from the floor. He is doing a well-rounded program that includes some cardio, strength training and a lot of stretching to loosen up his tight spots; he's well on the way to achieving his fitness and wellness goals even though at the start the stretching was difficult for him to do.

Most people want what's easy to do or prefer to do what they are good at; unfortunately often at the expense of exercises, activities or foods they really need. A balanced program will flush out weak links and imbalances in the body. It is common that many people need to do some exercises that are not easy for them as they target to improve the weak links. Hardly anyone is great at doing new exercises, therefore it is logical that these may not be your favorite. As muscles start to balance and weak links strengthen you will find that you start to enjoy the exercises, workouts or activity. So persevere - it does get easier.

STEP TWO - MATCH YOUR ACTIONS TO YOUR GOALS

QUICK TIPS

- Schedule at least 20-40 minutes for strength workouts, 10-30 minutes for cardiovascular (aerobic) training and 10 minutes of stretching 3 to 5 times per week depending on what goals you want to achieve, how quickly you want to achieve them, your age and your current physical health.

- If you have good general health with no injuries you may exercise or work out at an effort level of 50 to 70% (with 100% being your absolute maximum) for most activities. As you increase your fitness over the next few weeks you may then gradually increase the effort level to 80%, 90% and occasionally 100% effort.

- If you are over 35 years of age and have little or no physical exercise background or you have poor health you will need to get a good physical check-up from a doctor before exercising. Once approved to exercise or work out, exercise at 50% to 70% effort and follow any advice your doctor has given you.

Now, go to the next pages to get information on what activities align with the goals you have named for your body in Step One. By the time you're done you should have a good idea of what activities you should be focusing on to achieve your fitness goals as well as some information about the kinds of foods you should be eating.

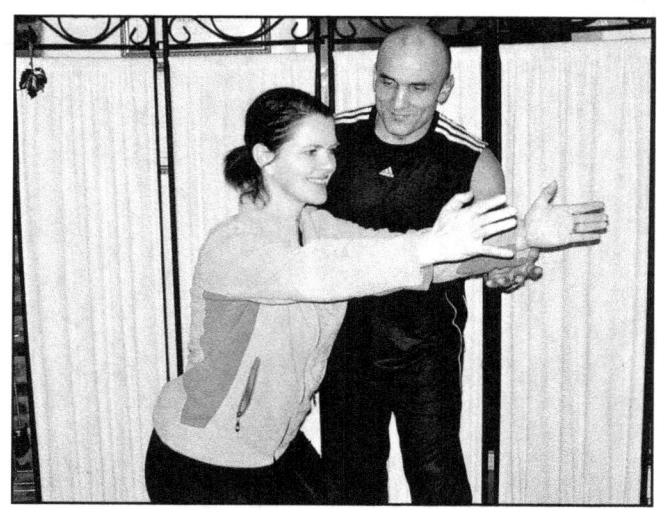

STEP TWO - MATCH YOUR ACTIONS TO YOUR GOALS

In this section you will find several charts. The first, Chart A, shows a variety of possible goals and the general activity types as well as diet and nutrition to achieve those goals. Charts B, C and D are a series of tables with more specific information about different activity types (strength, cardio and flexibility) while Chart E gives some food and diet basics.

Look over the following charts to see which actions match your fitness goals. Make a list on the blank page at the end of this step as you go through the charts of the actions that match your goals. Once you're done you should have a good idea of the activities to focus on for your goals.

CHART A - DO YOUR ACTIONS ACHIEVE YOUR GOALS?

SAMPLE GOALS	Strength Training ACTION	Cardio Workouts ACTION	Stretching ACTION	Diet, Nutrition, Food
Look Good	Yes	Yes	No	Yes
Be Healthy/ Energetic	Yes	Yes	Yes	Yes
Lose Body Fat	Yes	Yes	No	Yes
Lose Muscle	Yes, if overtraining	Yes, if overtraining	No	Too little food
Get Strong	Yes	Some	Some	Helps
Build Muscle	Yes	Some	Some	Helps
Look Sexy and Toned	Yes	Yes	Yes	Yes
Increase Metabolism	Yes	Yes	No	Yes
Cardio Fit	Yes	Yes	No	Helps
Rehabilitate Injury	Yes	Yes	Yes	Yes
Lower Metabolism	No	No	No	Too little food
Get Fat	No	No	No	Too much food
Get Stiff and Weak	No	No	No	Yes

STEP TWO - MATCH YOUR ACTIONS TO YOUR GOALS

CHART B - AEROBIC/CARDIO EXERCISES

ACTIVITY	Achieves Strength Goals	Achieves Cardio Goals	Achieves Stretch Goals	Comments on Metabolism and Calorie Expenditure
Cross country skiing	NO	YES	NO	Very high calorie burner. SPEEDS METABOLISM
Skip/sprint/run	NO	YES	NO	Very high calorie burner. SPEEDS METABOLISM
Jog/swim/bike/row	NO	YES	NO	Mid calorie burner. SPEEDS METABOLISM
Most team sports: soccer, football, etc.	NO	YES	NO	Very high calorie burner. SPEEDS METABOLISM
Brisk walking/hiking	NO	YES	NO	Mid calorie burner. SPEEDS METABOLISM
Racquetball/ handball, etc.	NO	YES	NO	Mid calorie burner. SPEEDS METABOLISM
Stepmill - moving staircase machine	NO	YES	NO	Very high calorie burner. SPEEDS METABOLISM
Stepper machine	NO	YES	NO	Mid to high calorie burner
Treadmill machine - running/jogging	NO	YES	NO	Very high calorie burner. SPEEDS METABOLISM
Bike/rower/elliptical machine	NO	YES	NO	Mid to high calorie burner

SAMPLE ACTIVITIES AND THE MAIN GOALS THEY ACHIEVE

Aerobic or cardio activities are those that last more than three minutes. They also involve many muscle groups at the same time. By increasing your aerobic fitness you can do more endurance activities with less effort and without getting out of breath.

Some home or commercial gym aerobic/cardio machines will work you harder than others. The Stairmaster Step-mill (rolling staircase) is a great example of one of the toughest machines. Next come the steppers and treadmill machines, then the cross-trainers, elliptical machines, rowers and bikes.

STEP TWO - MATCH YOUR ACTIONS TO YOUR GOALS

CHART C - STRENGTH TRAINING EXERCISES

ACTIVITY	Achieves Strength Goals	Achieves Cardio Goals	Achieves Stretch Goals	Comments on Metabolism and Calorie Expenditure
Body weight exercises	YES	YES	SOME	High intensity = higher calories burned. SPEEDS METABOLISM
Free weights: bars and dumbbells	YES	IN A CIRCUIT	SOME	High intensity = higher calories burned. SPEEDS METABOLISM
Strength machines or bands	YES	IN A CIRCUIT	SOME	High intensity = higher calories burned. SPEEDS METABOLISM

SAMPLE ACTIVITIES AND THE MAIN GOALS THEY ACHIEVE

There are many ways to do strength training. The three most common ways are: a) simple body weight exercises such as push-ups, pull-ups, crunches; b) free weights such as bench press, squats, dead-lifts and chin-ups; c) machines or bands such as bench press, squats or leg press, pull-downs and rows.

There are many different types of strength training from stability and endurance (high repetitions of 12 or more), hypertrophy - muscle building (medium repetitions of 6 to 12), strength (low repetitions of 1 to 6 with heavy weights) and power training (heavy weights, low repetitions done with speed).

CHART D - STRETCH/FLEXIBILITY WORKOUTS

ACTIVITY	Achieves Strength Goals	Achieves Cardio Goals	Achieves Stretch Goals	How Far to Stretch
Scientific Stretching	SOME	NO	YES	To the point of discomfort only
Yoga	SOME	NO	YES	To the point of discomfort only
Pilates	SOME	NO	YES	To the point of discomfort only

SAMPLE ACTIVITIES AND THE MAIN GOALS THEY ACHIEVE

Stretching is key to flexibility and is used to warm up and cool down the body before and after workouts or sport. It can help rehabilitate injured muscles and increase range of motion which helps prevent injuries. As the body ages it loses elasticity mostly due to inactivity. Stretch to regain elasticity and range of movement which also helps with balance, and agility, and reduces the chance of tearing stiff, shortened muscles.

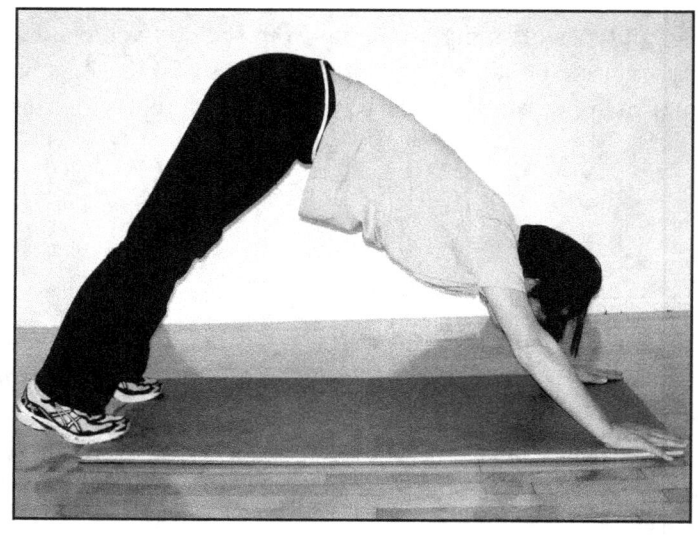

CHART E - FOOD AND DIET BASICS

Food and Diet Basics to Change Body	Eat Proteins	Eat Fats	Eat Carbohydrates
Maintain Current Body Condition	1 to 2g per kg of body weight/day	0.4g per kg of body weight/day	2 to 3g per kg of body weight/day
To Lose Weight (body fat) - Reduce or Burn 3500 to 7000 Calories/Week	Increase Protein	Low Fat	Low sugar and starches
To Gain Lean Muscle - Increase 700 to 1400 Calories/Week	Increase Protein	Medium Fat	Plenty of green and colored vegetables
To Increase Energy	Increase Protein	Medium Fat	Plenty of green and colored vegetables

According to the American College of Sports Medicine, the minimum recommended daily calorie consumption for women is 1200 to 1300. For men the minimum recommended daily calorie consumption is 1500 to 1800.

QUICK TIPS

By now you should have a list of activities that match your top three goals (from Step One). This is very important because this list will guide you towards your goals. Without it you're taking a gamble and could be wasting time, energy and possibly even money. Along with a list of activities that best fit your goals, you will also have some idea of what you need to do with your food (don't forget, food and exercise go together to get results) and diet. You will get a lot more information and advice about food and diet in "Step Seven - Diet Review".

Now that you have an idea of which activities to focus on, let's get you started! In the next section you will either do "Step 2A - For Currently Inactive People" (if you're not exercising right now) or "Step 2B - For Currently Inactive People" (if you're already working out and exercising). Go ahead, choose your step and continue with your personal fitness program.

STEP 2A - FOR CURRENTLY INACTIVE PEOPLE

If you are currently exercising or doing physical activity then skip this step and go directly to page 33 and do "Step 2B - For Currently Active People".

This step (Step 2A) is only for people who are not currently active or working out.

If you were active in the past and are not currently active or working out now, fill out the form below using the spaces provided to write your answers.

What fitness goals were you trying to achieve in the past? How long ago was this?

_____

What activities or type of workout were you doing in the past?

STRENGTH WORKOUTS_____(minutes/week) whether body weight, machine or free weight training.

CARDIO WORKOUTS_____(minutes/week) whether aerobic machines, e.g. tread-mill, bike, stepper etc., or outdoor jog, swim, cycle etc.

STRETCH WORKOUTS_____(minutes/week) whether yoga, pilates, scientific stretching or other.

OTHER ACTIVITIES OR WORKOUTS_____

How many workouts were you doing each week? (circle the answer that fits best)

1 to 2   2 to 3   3 to 5   Other_____

On average, what level of difficulty would you rate each workout? 100% being super hard, maximum effort. (circle the answer that fits best)

20 to 30%   40 to 50%   60 to 70%   80 to 90%

Over what duration did you do these workouts or activities?

1 to 3 months   3 to 6 months   6 to 12 months   Other_____

What percentage of your fitness goals did you attain doing the above workouts?

40 to 50%   50 to 60%   60 to 70%   70 to 80%   80 to 90%   Other_____

If you did not achieve 100% of your goals, why not?_____

_____

STEP 2A - FOR CURRENTLY INACTIVE PEOPLE

QUICK TIPS

- Write down the goals you decided on from "Step One - Name Your Goals" and when you want to achieve them. Put them somewhere you will see them every day to remind yourself where you're heading.

- Review "Step Two - Match Actions to Goals" Charts A and B and write down which activities match your fitness goals.

- Examples of a wrongly matched activity to goal: a silly one would be to practice swimming in order to run a marathon. A less obvious example would be going for walks or doing aerobics classes in the hope that it will make you strong and toned (the correct activity to increase strength and tone would be real strength training, not cardio training).

- **Start exercising at about 50 to 70% effort** if you are not injured and you're in good health. Gradually increase the effort when it gets too easy. This will speed up your progress and help get you to your goals safely and quickly.

- Use large muscle groups in exercises, such as legs, back and chest, to stir up your metabolism.

- **The body is as strong as its weakest link.** For example, a weak grip means poor back training because you won't be able to hold onto a bar in order to do exercises like pull-ups that work the back. To strengthen your back you will need to strengthen your grip as well.

- **The body is as flexible as its tightest spot.** For example, you try to stretch the back of your legs (hamstrings) but you mostly feel the tightness in your calf muscles. To access and stretch your hamstrings you will also need to stretch or lengthen your calf muscles.

- If you are new to exercise start out at an easy pace. Focus on correct form first. Even when you start out gently and gradually increase effort or workload (weight or resistance) you will often find hidden weak links in your body that have been lying dormant for years. These will start to surface as you exercise regularly. Don't worry, this is a good thing as now you can do something about it before any real or serious damage or injury occurs under future stress during living, sport or when on vacation.

- Now go on to "Risk Assessment" on page 37. Fill out the Physical Activity Readiness Questionnaire (PAR-Q).

"I have not failed. I've just found 10,000 ways that won't work." **Thomas Edison**

STEP 2B - FOR CURRENTLY ACTIVE PEOPLE

If you already did "Step 2A - For Currently Inactive People" you will not do this section but will go directly on to page 37.

This section is only for people who are already active and working out.

STEP 2B - FOR CURRENTLY ACTIVE PEOPLE

If you are currently active and working out, fill out the form below to better analyze whether or not what you are doing will really achieve your fitness goals. Write your answers to the following questions in the spaces provided in this book below.

What fitness goals are you trying to achieve?

_____

What activities or type of workout are you currently doing?

STRENGTH WORKOUTS_____(minutes/week) whether body weight, machine or free weight training.

CARDIO WORKOUTS_____(minutes/week) whether aerobic machines e.g. treadmill, bike, stepper etc. or aerobic classes, outdoor jog, swim, cycle etc.

STRETCH WORKOUTS_____(minutes/week) whether yoga, pilates, scientific stretching or other.

OTHER ACTIVITIES OR SPORTS_____ (minutes/week)

How many workouts are you doing each week? (circle the answer that fits best)

1 to 2   2 to 3   3 to 5   Other

On average, what level of difficulty would you rate each workout? 100% being super hard, maximum effort. (circle the answer that fits best)

20 to 30%   40 to 50%   60 to 70%   80 to 90%

How long have you been doing these workouts or activities?

1 to 3 months   3 to 6 months   6 to 12 months   Other_____

What percentage of your fitness goals do you feel you have already attained doing the above workouts?

40 to 50%   50 to 60%   60 to 70%   70 to 80%   80 to 90%   Other_____

If you haven't achieved 100% of your goals yet, why not?_____

_____

STEP 2B - FOR CURRENTLY ACTIVE PEOPLE

If you haven't achieved your goals yet even though you have been working out, below are a few situations you might find yourself in:

- If you have been working out for a few months but notice little or no results, go back to STEP TWO - MATCH ACTIONS TO GOALS CHARTS A & B and review the information. It is possible you are not doing the correct activities to reach your goals.
- If your current workouts do not include the three basics; strength, cardio and flexibility then they are unbalanced and need to be improved. It's likely this is inhibiting getting results.
- To be considered active one should be doing 2 to 4 workouts per week at home, at the gym or playing some sport.
- If you are doing the right activity for your goals, what about frequency, duration, intensity, effort, form and technique? Are you over-training or under-training? These are all key factors. Don't forget nutrition and diet, which are also key to getting results.

You may find yourself having to change your current activity, exercise or workout to align to your goals. Perhaps you only need to refine, adjust, change or improve a little on what you are already doing to speed up your progress to fully attain your fitness goals.

QUICK TIPS
- *Basics:* Challenge your strength, breathing and flexibility at least 2 to 3 times per week.
- *Prepare:* Don't skip warm-ups and cool downs.
- *Aerobic fitness:* Do something that gets you out of breath at least 2 to 3 times per week by jogging, swimming or cycling or other such aerobic activity.
- *Strength fitness:* Do a minimum of 2-3 strength workouts per week by lifting something heavier than what you are used to. Challenge yourself.
- *Stretch fitness:* Do 2-3 stretch workouts per week.
- *Rest:* Alternate workouts; Day 1 is strength day, Day 2 is cardio and stretching and so on.
- *Stiff lower back:* Stretch every morning upon waking and throughout the day as needed.
- *Abs:* Pull your abs in a few minutes a day as you walk, sit or stand.
- *Track:* Log what you do - length of time, quality and effort level. Write down your workouts, diet, body measurements, strength, etc. Measure and record what you want to improve.

CORRECT ACTIVITY ALIGNED & APPLIED TO GOAL = RESULTS!

Go on to "Risk Assessment" on page 37 and fill out the PAR-Q (Physical Activity Readiness Questionnaire)

RISK ASSESSMENT - BEFORE YOU START

Physical Activity Readiness Questionnaire (PAR-Q)

The American College of Sports Medicine recommends you see a doctor if any of the following applies: you are a man older than 45 or a woman older than 55, you have a family history of heart disease before age 55, you have high blood pressure, cholesterol, you smoke, you are overweight or obese.

The purpose of the PAR-Q is to assess any potential risk factors before starting any vigorous activity or workouts. If you answer yes to one or more of the questions seek medical advice before starting any exercise or diet program.

NAME:		AGE:	DATE:

Regular exercise is associated with many health benefits, yet any change of activity may increase the risk of injury. Completion of this questionnaire is a first step when planning to increase the amount of physical activity in your life. Please read each question carefully and answer every question honestly.

Yes	No	1) Has a physician ever said you have a heart condition and you should only do physical activity recommended by a physician?
Yes	No	2) When you do physical activity, do you feel pain in your chest?
Yes	No	3) Have you had chest pain in the past month when you were not doing physical activity?
Yes	No	4) Do you ever lose consciousness or do you lose your balance because of dizziness?
Yes	No	5) Do you have a joint or bone problem that may be made worse by a change in your physical activity?
Yes	No	6) Is a physician currently prescribing medications for your blood pressure or heart condition?
Yes	No	7) Are you pregnant?
Yes	No	8) Do you have insulin-dependent diabetes?
Yes	No	9) Are you 69 years of age or older and not used to being very active?
Yes	No	Do you know of any other reason you should not exercise or increase your physical activity?

IMPORTANT NOTE: If you answered yes to any of the above questions, talk with your doctor BEFORE you start any vigorous physical activity. Tell you doctor your intent to exercise and to which questions you answered yes. If you honestly answered no to all questions you can be reasonably positive that you can safely increase your level of physical activity gradually. At a later date if your health changes so you then answer yes to any of the above questions, seek guidance from a physician.

Now that you have named your goals, learned which activities will best achieve them and have a few tips for getting started, go on to the next step, "Step Three – Obstacles". There you will identify things that can get in the way of your success, slow you down, or discourage you, and you'll also learn how to overcome these things to get the body you want faster.

"Without self-discipline, success is impossible, period." Lou Holtz

STEP THREE - OBSTACLES

STEP THREE - OBSTACLES

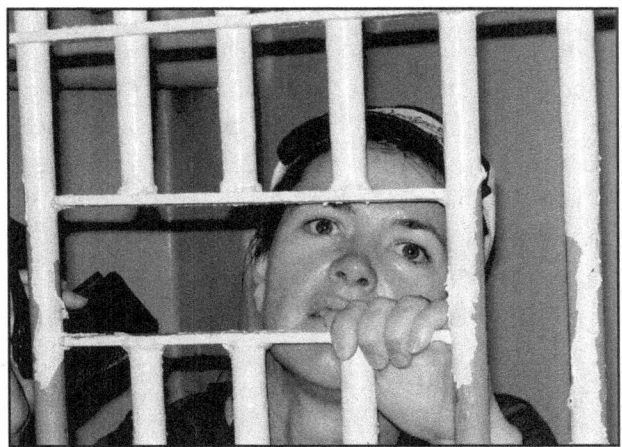

Whenever anyone tries to achieve a worthwhile goal you can bet that there will also be problems and obstacles that will need to be overcome along the way. It's a good idea to be prepared and have a strategy in place to overcome as many as possible of these problems or barriers as they occur.

Below are four of the more common barriers, obstacles or problems I have observed over my more than 20 years of working professionally and helping people achieve their fitness goals. Interestingly, they aren't things someone else puts there to stop you. Most often, the common ones are self-created.

BEWARE OF THE FOUR COMMON OBSTACLES OR BARRIERS TO SUCCESS!

1. WEAK INTEREST - When someone lacks a strong desire to achieve goals.
2. DON'T KNOW - When a person simply doesn't know what to do, when to do it or how to do it.
3. FALSE INFORMATION - When a person is operating from incorrect and false information that he thinks is correct. The problem is that results are hard to come by and there is a high probability of injury.
4. THE "KNOW-ALL" WITH THE CLOSED MIND - When a person already "knows it all" and is unwilling to learn anything new. The mind is closed.

We will now take a look at each obstacle and you can work out what your own potential obstacles to success are. Knowing these opens the door to overcoming them – you can't win a battle against an enemy you can't see and don't know is there.

WEAK INTEREST

The first obstacle to achieving great success is the *lack of strong desire or interest* in wanting to really achieve those goals. The higher your interest level, the more motivated and committed you will be to achieving your goals. The higher the priority you set for your goals, the more willing you will be to make changes and get into action. This is the key to the level of success you will achieve. Mental strength always comes before focused physical actions. **Any action in the physical world is always preceded by an idea, thought or decision. Do not underestimate your most vital and potent tool: your own mind. Use it well.**

SUCCESS TRIANGLE - THREE STEPS TO SUCCESS

1. INTEREST LEVEL IS HIGH
2. 100% COMMITTED TO GOALS
3. RIGHT ACTIONS ARE TAKEN

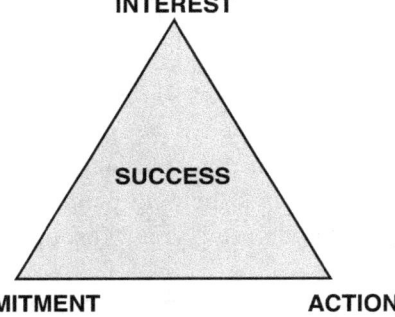

SUCCESS: Achievement of intention; the achievement of something planned or attempted.

INTEREST: Involvement; somebody's involvement with something that makes its progress or success important to him or her.

COMMITMENT: A loyalty; a devotion or dedication, e.g. to a cause, person or relationship.

ACTION: Doing something toward a goal; the process of doing something in order to achieve a purpose.

SOURCE OF DEFINITIONS: http://encarta.msn.com/dictionary

All three items belonging to each corner of the Success Triangle must be present if success is to occur. Each corner affects the others. If any one corner is weak it will affect or lower the other two corners. If one corner is very strong it will help lift the other two corners. For example, if someone is only partially interested in achieving weight loss (say, because a spouse told them to do it) they are unlikely to be very committed to the program or put much effort or action into reaching that goal.

DON'T KNOW

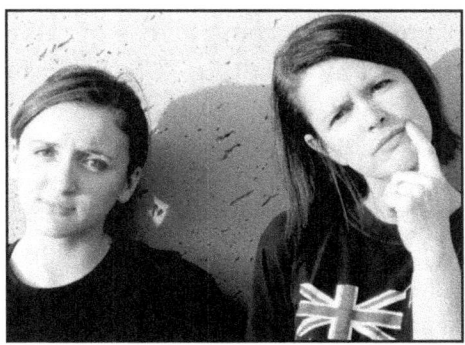

If you have no idea or information on how to lose weight, build muscle, get fit or eat right that would obviously pose a problem or create an obstacle or barrier to achieving your fitness goals.

Few people know much about health & fitness, let alone the real basic truths of food, diet, exercise and workouts. *This is the most common of all obstacles* and affects the majority of people trying to achieve fitness goals. Getting the right know-how will, when applied, consistently achieve results.

Some of the more common reasons for exercise or program failing to get good, lasting results are:

- Workout inefficiency (wasting time)
- Incorrect program or activity (not doing the right actions)
- Poor exercise form and technique execution (not doing it properly)
- Lack of exercise frequency and intensity (not doing enough)

I have observed that most people who are getting some results are doing so at a working rate of about 40-50% efficiency. That means they are still wasting 50-60% of their time because of poor exercise form, type, frequency, effort, program, sequence etc. OK, what about the rest who are getting very little improvement or results? What percentage of time are they wasting?

Don't waste your time, money, effort and possibly your health. Make sure you get the correct knowledge to do it right and get great results.

Truthfully, this obstacle is easy to overcome because someone who can admit he or she doesn't know isn't impeded by the false belief that he or she *does* know. Just continue through this book, learning and applying the correct information to achieve specific fitness and wellness goals. So, if you are someone with this obstacle, rest assured, you're in the right place and very soon you will have this one licked for good!

FALSE INFORMATION

Here are two classic examples I've come across of false information: "Walking is the best form of exercise and is a great way to get fit." "To build muscle you need to eat a lot of food." The truths are: walking is a low-calorie-burning activity that *will not* get you fit and eating a lot will build fat, *not* muscle. To build muscle you *must* do strength training.

False information on fitness is one of the most common obstacles that plague people and it has many non-optimum ramifications. The obvious solution is to simply get the *right* fitness information from credible sources (not your hairdresser, your friend in the gym or your favorite TV personality), so that when you apply it exactly you get the results you want.

A test of whether information is correct is how well it helps the majority of people most of the time. Watch out for tricky, gimmicky marketing (you'll see infomercials on TV rife with false information) that state things like, "The 4 minute-a-day miracle workout!" "The ultimate abs gadget that 'guarantees results in 10 days' or your money back." "The miracle cure diet; lose 10 pounds of fat in 2 weeks." The list goes on and on.

A symptom that people are using false information is they get few or no lasting results. They might appear to be in better shape for a while, but in six month's, very often they are in even worse shape than when they started.

As a professional trainer and exercise enthusiast I have observed that people with the Second and Third Obstacles fail to get good results. Their workouts are inefficient and they have poor exercise form. This is obviously a large waste of time, effort and money. There are those who are getting some results but they are doing so at about 40 to 50% workout efficiency, which means they are still wasting half their time with poor exercise form, choice, program or sequence. Imagine if they knew how to increase their efficiency!

The good news is that people are trying to do something about their health and fitness. What a difference to safety, efficiency and results it would make if they only went to a little further trouble to find, learn and put into practice some of the true key basics of fitness. By choosing this book you have taken a very important step in the right direction to ensure you get correct information and learn how to use it properly.

THE "KNOW-ALL"

This is the closed-minded person who thinks he knows it all and has all the answers to everything. Unfortunately the "Know-All" knows very little and has shut down his own learning capacity. The truth is that the very best fitness professionals never believe they know it all and are always eager to learn more to get even better results for themselves and their clients. The following are some characteristics you may find in the "Know-All":

1. They sound authoritative when they speak and if challenged will get quite upset

2. They are quick to dispense "expert opinions" on topics they are not expert in

3. They most likely got their information from fitness or muscle magazines, books, articles, friends, associates or some random website. This makes them "expert"

4. They "know all about food, diet, exercise and fitness", the only problem is that they are getting little or no lasting results, despite all they "know"

5. They don't know that they don't know

6. They are unable to really look, listen and learn. Try to teach them something new and they'll reject it or argue with you

7. They are difficult to help. They come up asking a professional for advice only to then reject it, telling you they already know it to the point of argument

8. If a new scientific cutting-edge, state-of-the-art piece of fitness information comes their way they cannot absorb it as their mind is shut off and unreceptive. Data goes straight on by

I am sure nobody reading this book is a "Know All", but if you do find yourself heading in that direction, keep in mind that it is a step in wisdom for a person to know what he knows and to also know what he doesn't know and to be willing to observe and test new data or information to see if it works. This is the correct view or attitude to have in order to get the most out of this book.

SOME SOLUTIONS TO OBSTACLES

It is true that in life things can and do pop up that get in the way of your best efforts to achieve a goal. It's very rare to find a person who hasn't had things come up to stop his forward progress. The important thing is to be aware of what can potentially get in your way and make sure you have some kind of a plan of how to overcome whatever slows you down or tries to stop you.

1. First think of obstacles you have personally experienced in the past when attempting to achieve fitness or weight-loss goals. Then think of any other obstacles that might get in your way either now or in the near future. Some examples could be an upcoming vacation, holidays, starting a new job, having a baby, having to work around young children, or whatever is real to you as an obstacle.

2. The next step is to think of a few bright ideas on how you plan to overcome any of these obstacles, especially if they already exist and are getting in your way or may in the future. My wife had the obstacle of working long hours and overcame this by setting time aside every evening to exercise no matter what, even if only for half an hour. Before she knew it her energy levels were way up and it became easier and easier to get those workouts in.

Naming your obstacles and how you can solve them are great tools and without a doubt will highly increase your potential success rate and prepare you to overcome any obstacles that may turn up.

Another good strategy is to simply recognize that anything that gets in the way of achieving your goals is an obstacle. Treat it the same as you would a mosquito trying to bite your arm.

Allowing obstacles or problems to appear, persist, stay and take control without any immediate action will result in slowed progress, stops, loss of hope, poor results, failures, or just plain old giving up.

Every problem, barrier or obstacle has a solution. One just needs to find it or come up with a bright idea. Doing this exercise now, before even beginning your fitness and wellness program, gets you proactive and will ensure greater success.

On the next page is the "Name the Obstacle, Name the Solution" chart. Fill it out using the thoughts you had about obstacles in the two steps above. Remember, you want to know in advance what can potentially get in your way and have a solution ready so you can treat obstacles as the "mosquitoes" they are to your goals.

NAME THE OBSTACLE, NAME THE SOLUTION

Name the Obstacle:

Name the Solution:

Name the Obstacle:

Name the Solution:

Name the Obstacle:

Name the Solution:

Name the Obstacle:

Name the Solution:

Name the Obstacle:

Name the Solution:

"When defeat comes, accept it as a signal that your plans are not sound, rebuild those plans, and set sail once more toward your coveted goal." Napoleon Hill

"The secret of success is constancy to purpose." Benjamin Disraeli

STEP FOUR - SUCCESS AND FAILURE

STEP FOUR - SUCCESS AND FAILURE

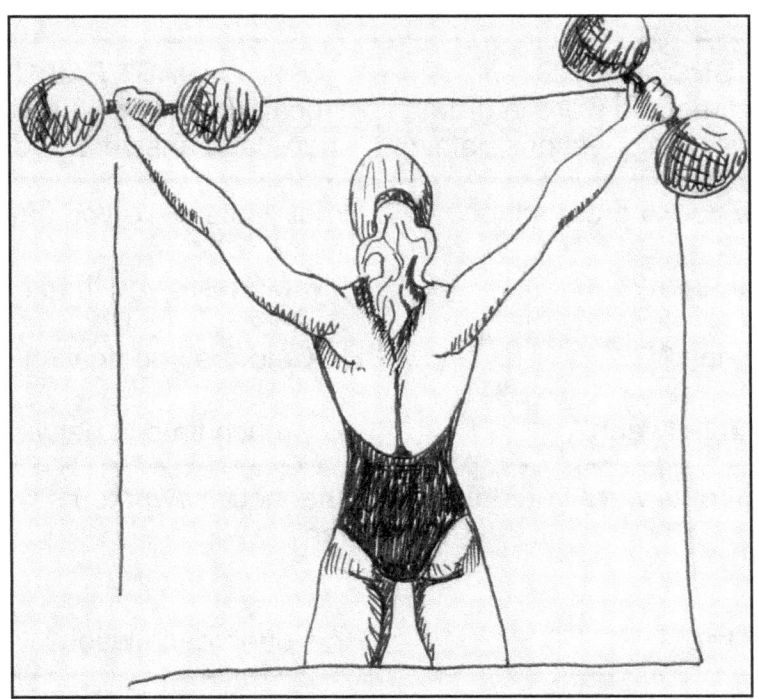

The purpose of this section is to review any time in the past you were in great shape to see what you were eating, how you were exercising and what kind of overall mental attitude you might have had that contributed to this condition. We want to find out if you can implement any of these past successful actions in the present to recreate the great results you got in the past.

Of course, there might be some variables that could limit you now that time has passed: your current age (if you're much older now your metabolism will have changed considerably), your current physical condition (if you've been ill for some time or sedentary for a long time) and your overall health and fitness levels.

Fill out the table below then continue to the next page:

PAST SUCCESSES Recall the last time you were in great shape and answer the questions below:	PAST FAILURES Recall when you were last really out of shape and answer the questions below:
What years were you in great shape? How old were you then? How old are you now? How much time in between?	What years were you out of shape? How old were you then? How old are you now? How much time in between?
What activity/workouts were you doing then? How often each week?	What activity/workouts were you doing then? How often each week?
What was your diet like? Number of meals per day?	What was your diet like? Number of meals per day?
What was your attitude like?	What was your attitude like?
What were your fitness goals?	What were your fitness goals?
Were you smoking or drinking alcohol? How often? Any medications?	Were you smoking or drinking alcohol? How often? Any medications?

Now, summarize your past successes and failures in the table below:

Past Successes	Past Failures
Activity (what were you doing physically)? Time elapsed since then?	Activity (what were you doing physically)? Time elapsed since then?
What were you doing with food and diet?	What were you doing with food and diet?
What was your mental attitude?	What was your mental attitude?

STEP FOUR - SUCCESS AND FAILURE

By comparing past successes and failures you should clearly see what worked in the past and what failed. Then take a look to see if you are able to repeat some or all of your past successes to do with exercise, food and attitude. The concept is that if you put those same past successes into action again, you should get similar results. The information in the failures section is also useful as it gives clues about what didn't work in the past and so what to avoid in your quest for health and fitness.

An exception regarding past success is that time has elapsed and possibly many things have changed since then. You may be a little or a lot older, your health might be worse than it was. Perhaps you've had injuries since then or perhaps your past successful activity is totally inappropriate for you now (maybe you played college football or basketball which wouldn't work if you're a sixty-five year-old grandfather with a knee replacement and a bad lower back).

FACTORS THAT WILL AFFECT REGAINING GREAT PHYSICAL CONDITION

TIME: the more time that has gone by in years, the harder it gets to replicate an earlier condition of great physical fitness.

EXERCISE HISTORY: how active or inactive you've been since you were last in great shape will affect results. If you've continued to be active you will find it easier to get back into great shape. If you've been inactive you'll have to get used to activity again so it might take a little longer. You've probably heard the saying, "Use it or lose it."

DIET: how good, bad or ugly your diet has been since your past great physical condition will also affect results. Eating food with poor nutritional value puts a large strain on the body; your liver might not be in the shape it once was or perhaps your heart has taken a "beating" with lots of high-fat, high-calorie fast food.

HEALTH HISTORY: your current or past surgeries and any debilitating illnesses will affect results.

POOR METABOLISM: if you slowed down your metabolism with poor diet and lack of physical activity this will affect results.

CURRENT LEVEL OF INTEREST IN ACHIEVING YOUR GOALS: how interested you are in achieving your fitness goals will most definitely affect the results you get.

Keep these factors in mind when you review what worked for you in the past. They can be worked around and perhaps you will have to do a few things differently, but it is a great exercise to take a look back to see how you were operating when you were doing well and were in good shape.

"Knowing is not enough; we must apply. Willing is not enough; we must do." Johann Wolfgang von Goethe

STEP FIVE - SCHEDULE FOR SUCCESS

STEP FIVE - SCHEDULE FOR SUCCESS

TICK, TOCK, TICK, TOCK, time is ticking, no time for procrastination. Do it... Go fit now!

To really be successful and achieve the goals you have set, you'll need to schedule *when* to do your workouts. Planning them out in advance will give them an importance they might not otherwise have and it will help ensure you keep moving toward your goals.

Go ahead now and fill out the following worksheet then use it to get started on your way to success.

SCHEDULE YOUR WORKOUTS

Fill out the Schedule Box below, stating which days you plan to do your strength, aerobic and stretch workouts along with any active sports activities.

SCHEDULE BOX

Monday	Tuesday	Wednesday	Thursday	Friday	Sat and Sun

QUICK TIPS

- *CHANGES:* The sooner you start making changes and aligning activities and food to your goals, the sooner you will get results.

- *DECISION:* If you haven't already done so, decide 100% that you really want to achieve your goals.

- *PRIORITIZE:* Decide right now to give top priority to your fitness goals.

- *SCHEDULE FOOD AND EXERCISE:* Get a journal and schedule in your food and workouts - when you intend to eat, drink and do exercise. Then once the food has been consumed or the workout done, write that fact down so you have a running record to track what's going into your body and what's going out. This is a powerful and insightful tool for success. Keeping a journal to schedule workouts will put you in greater control.

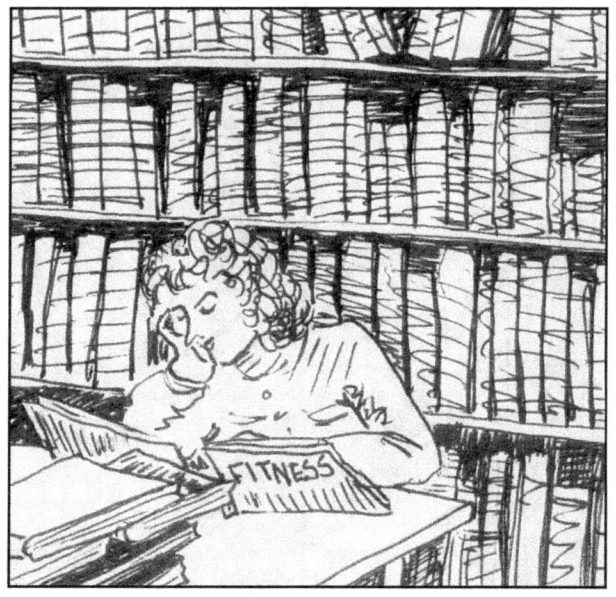

Correct knowledge correctly applied creates a
powerful condition. If possible, learn something
new on a daily basis and learn as much as you
can.

"The ability to convert ideas to things is the secret to outward success."

Henry Ward Beecher

STEP SIX - TO-DO LIST

This step is very important as you will put together the earlier steps and organize them as a whole to ensure you make your goals an actuality.

ACTION PLAN FOR THE FIRST ONE TO EIGHT WEEKS

WEEKS 1 to 8: Start date:_____Finish date:_____

GOALS: WHAT DO YOU WANT TO ACHIEVE in the first eight weeks?

WHAT ACTIVITIES ARE RECOMMENDED FOR YOUR GOALS :

STRENGTH   CARDIO   STRETCHING

HOW MANY WORKOUTS EACH WEEK: 1 to 2   3 to 4   5 to 6

EFFORT LEVEL: 2-4 out of 10, 5-7 out of 10, 8-10 out of 10 (10 being most effort)

SCHEDULED TIME FOR WORKOUTS/ACTIVITIES

ACTIVITY	Mon	Tues	Wed	Thurs	Fri	Sat/Sun
Strength Workouts	Time:	Time:	Time:	Time:	Time:	Time:
Cardio Workouts	Time:	Time:	Time:	Time:	Time:	Time:
Stretch Workouts	Time:	Time:	Time:	Time:	Time:	Time:

ANY DIETARY CHANGES NEEDED OR RECOMMENDED?

1. Change or improve:_____

2. Change or improve:_____

3. Change or improve:_____

THE NEXT EIGHT WEEKS

Do the worksheet on this page AFTER completing the first eight weeks. Once you reach your initial goals you'll find there might be new goals to name and reach for. Make sure you look at what worked and what needs improving.

WEEKS 9 to 16: Start date:_____ Finish date:_____

GOALS: WHAT DO YOU WANT TO ACHIEVE in the next eight weeks?

WHAT ACTIVITIES ARE RECOMMENDED FOR YOUR GOALS :

STRENGTH   CARDIO   STRETCHING

HOW MANY WORKOUTS EACH WEEK: 1 to 2   3 to 4   5 to 6

EFFORT LEVEL: 2-4 out of 10, 5-7 out of 10, 8-10 out of 10 (10 being most effort)

SCHEDULED TIME FOR WORKOUTS/ACTIVITIES

ACTIVITY	Mon	Tues	Wed	Thurs	Fri	Sat/Sun
Strength Workouts	Time:	Time:	Time:	Time:	Time:	Time:
Cardio Workouts	Time:	Time:	Time:	Time:	Time:	Time:
Stretch Workouts	Time:	Time:	Time:	Time:	Time:	Time:

ANY DIETARY CHANGES NEEDED OR RECOMMENDED?

1. Change or improve:_____

2. Change or improve:_____

3. Change or improve:_____

FORMULA FOR FITNESS SUCCESS:

GOALS + RIGHT ACTIVITY + RIGHT NUTRITION = RESULTS

"Let food be your medicine and medicine be your food." Hippocrates

"Don't dig your grave with your own knife and fork." English Proverb

STEP SEVEN - DIET REVIEW

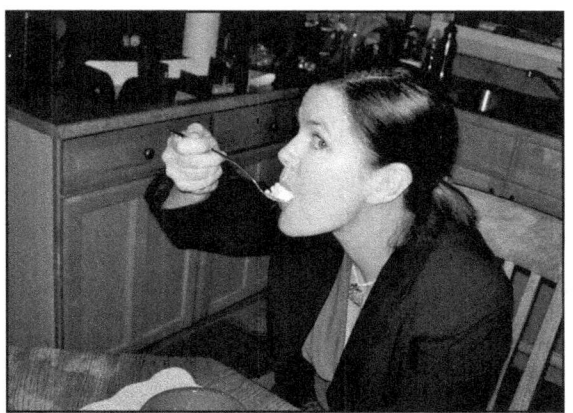

*You need not deny yourself treats as long as
there is some moderation.*

EAT FOR PURPOSE

Well, we've all heard the saying, "You are what you eat." There is some truth in that statement when it comes to the human body. If you follow the tips in this section you will have a better chance of success if your goal is to be healthier, more energetic or to reduce body fat.

Make it a priority to eat for purpose - food should:
1. Be nutritious
2. Aid your fitness goals
3. Be tasty

The trick is to see how you can have nutritious food that achieves your goals while being as tasty as possible. If you don't eat for purpose your long-term plans of achieving your health and fitness goals will be a very difficult task to attain.

Many people only eat for taste, flavor and enjoyment; this is O.K., except that it may or may not be nutritious. Even worse, the food could be outright dangerous and detrimental to your health. Observe the escalating numbers of weight related diseases such as:

- *Heart disease* - heart attack, congestive heart failure, sudden cardiac death, angina (lack of blood causing chest pain and a feeling of suffocation), stroke (ruptured blood vessel in the brain), high blood pressure or blood cholesterol
- *Diabetes type 2* (diet related)
- *Osteoarthritis* (degenerative joint disease)
- *Complications* of pregnancy, menstrual irregularities, infertility, irregular ovulation, incontinence and more.

QUICK GLANCE DIET REVIEW AND TIPS

Answer the questions in Column A and compare with tips in Column B.

COLUMN A	COLUMN B
How many servings of white processed sugary foods or snacks do you have in your daily diet? E.g. Sodas, candy, donuts etc.	**SUGAR:** Cut out all processed SUGAR. That is; refined, white & processed. Eat some fruits, use the Glycemic Index (GI) on page 77 to choose low GI foods.
When do you eat your largest meal of the day? Beginning of the day End of the day	**INVERTED PYRAMID:** Eat largest meals in the morning or at lunch & the smallest meals at night.
Do you ever skip breakfast? YES NO	**SKIPPED BREAKFAST:** Do not skip breakfast; it kick-starts your energy and speeds up metabolism for the day.
Do you eat large food portions? YES NO	**PORTION SIZE:** For weight loss, reduce size of all meals. Leave some on your plate at each meal.
How many times a day do you eat and snack? 1 2 3 4 5 6 7 8 other_____	**EAT MULTIPLE SMALL MEALS:** Eat small to medium sized meals or snacks every 3-4 hours. No snacking in between to rest stomach. Gradually reduce size of meals towards nightfall.
Do you <u>all</u> your meals and snacks contain some protein and fat? YES NO	**BALANCE MEALS & SNACKS:** All meals & snacks must include proteins, fats and carbohydrates.
How many cups of water do you drink per day? _____	**WATER:** Drink 8 to 12 (8 ounce glasses) per day.
Do you drink alcohol or smoke cigarettes? YES NO IF YES HOW MUCH?	**AVOID EMPTY CALORIES:** Alcoholic beverages are useless, empty calories & operate as simple sugars. Cigarettes reduce lung capacity.
Do you take daily vitamins and minerals and some healthy oil? YES NO	**TAKE DAILY VITAMINS, MINERALS & OIL:** Take a daily multi vitamin/mineral supplement. Include flax seed oil or similar.
What percentage of your daily meals come from natural versus processed foods? PROCESSED – made by man _____% Sodas, diet products, cereals, canned foods, gum, microwave products etc NATURAL – grown by nature _____% Fruits, vegetables, fish, chicken, eggs etc.	**AVOID PROCESSED FOOD:** Avoid greasy, oily, fried, creamy & high saturated fat (animal) foods. **PROCESSED,** Aspartame-filled, sugary, buttery foods. AVOID: alcohol, diet foods, drinks, sodas, gum, artificial sugar replacement, etc. GO AS NATURAL AS YOU CAN. See website www.NewsTarget.com for good information
Are you on any psychiatric, anti-depressant, bipolar, ADHD or other psychotropic medication? YES NO	**AVOID PSYCHOTROPIC DRUGS:** Find out the real side effects and what nutrients are being robbed from your body. Seek a natural practitioner for natural cures. Also visit http://www.cchr.org for more information.

Once you have compared your answers with the tips in Column B, make changes to your diet based on those tips and the tips (below) from the Eat Smart Pyramid and the Quick Food Tips section.

EAT SMART PYRAMID

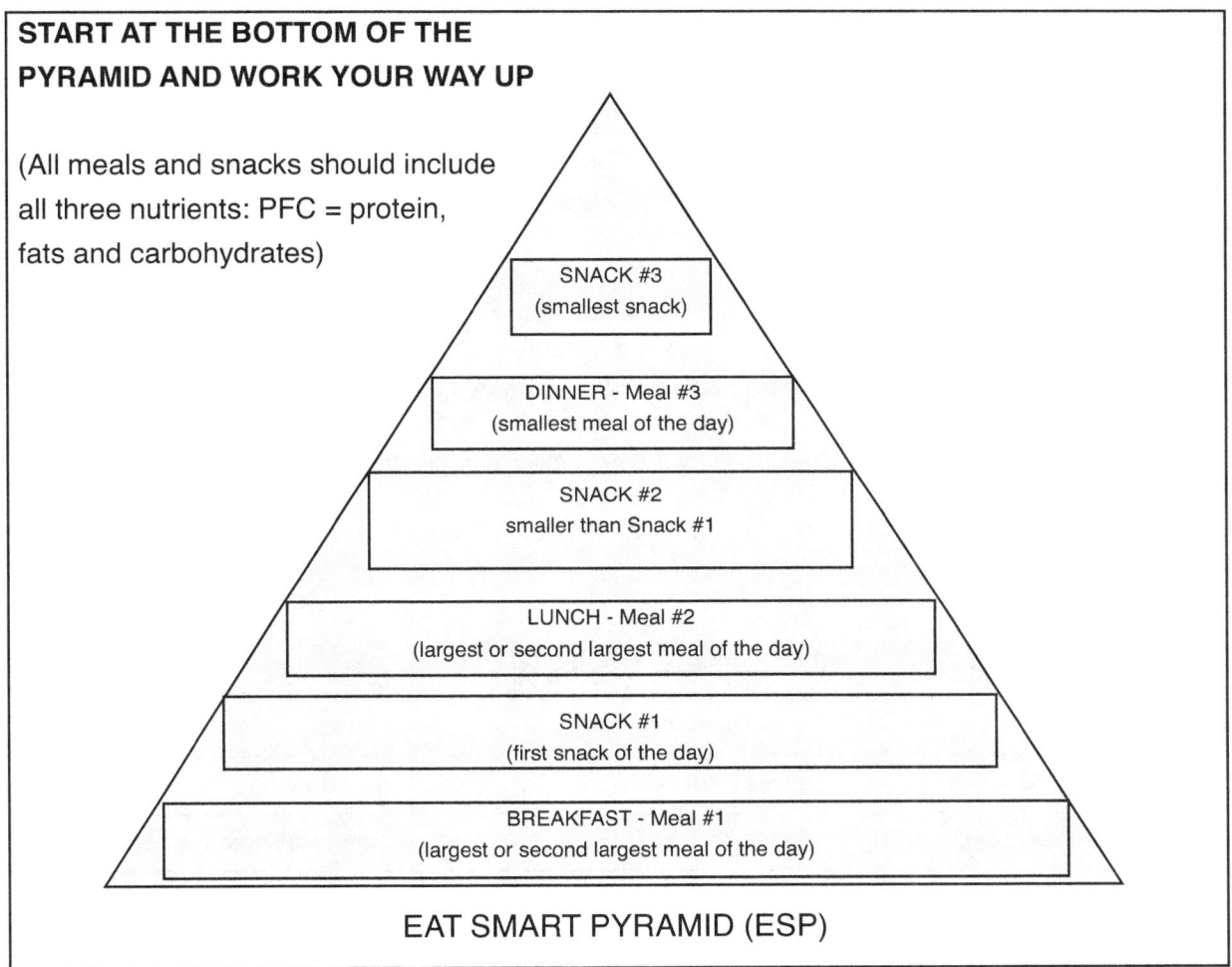

START AT THE BOTTOM OF THE PYRAMID AND WORK YOUR WAY UP

(All meals and snacks should include all three nutrients: PFC = protein, fats and carbohydrates)

SNACK #3
(smallest snack)

DINNER - Meal #3
(smallest meal of the day)

SNACK #2
smaller than Snack #1

LUNCH - Meal #2
(largest or second largest meal of the day)

SNACK #1
(first snack of the day)

BREAKFAST - Meal #1
(largest or second largest meal of the day)

EAT SMART PYRAMID (ESP)

Examples of high-quality protein, carbohydrates and fats:
PROTEIN - lean protein
CARBOHYDRATES - fresh vegetables
FATS - vegetable fats (just a little)

EAT SMART PYRAMID FOOD TIPS

At the bottom of the pyramid is the start of the day. This is when you have the whole day ahead of you. So this is a good time to eat up; ideally eat the largest meal of the day in the morning. If you can't do this, make your next meal (lunch) or morning snack the largest of the day.

As the day comes to a close the pyramid gets smaller. This indicates that you should eat less and smaller portions at night or as the day ends. The reason behind this is that most people are less active and are winding down at the end of the day so the body needs less fuel. "Eat for the oncoming event" is a fair diet motto. Are you more active today? Eat a little more. Less activity equals less food needed. If you are going to be sedentary all day eat less. If you are going hiking, then eat a little more as you will need more calories (fuel) to sustain you through the hike.

Beware of any "expert" or doctor who tells you not to exercise as part of your weight-loss program. If you diet only (only reduce calorie intake) the weight loss will also come from lean tissue (muscle). No fad diets are needed for any long term success. Use simple time-proven workable know-how on food; add some willingness to make changes, a touch of discipline to keep control and focus on your goals and you will be a winner, achieving your fitness goals sooner than you think.

Recording your daily food habits is a great way to help you control and make improvements to your diet.

PROTEINS	CARBOHYDRATES	FATS
egg white	vegetables, dark leafy greens	olives
egg yolk (in moderation)	some fresh fruit	avocado
fish (white and oily) e.g. tuna	brown rice	flaxseeds, sesame seeds
lean chicken (grilled, not fried)	oatmeal	nuts - almonds, cashews etc
veal (grilled, not fried)	quinoa	fish oil, olive oil, flaxseed oil
tofu and soy products	beans	seeds - sunflower, pumpkin etc
protein powder (whey, soy)	salads	coconut oil
beans e.g. navy, black, kidney	barley	

EAT SMART PYRAMID

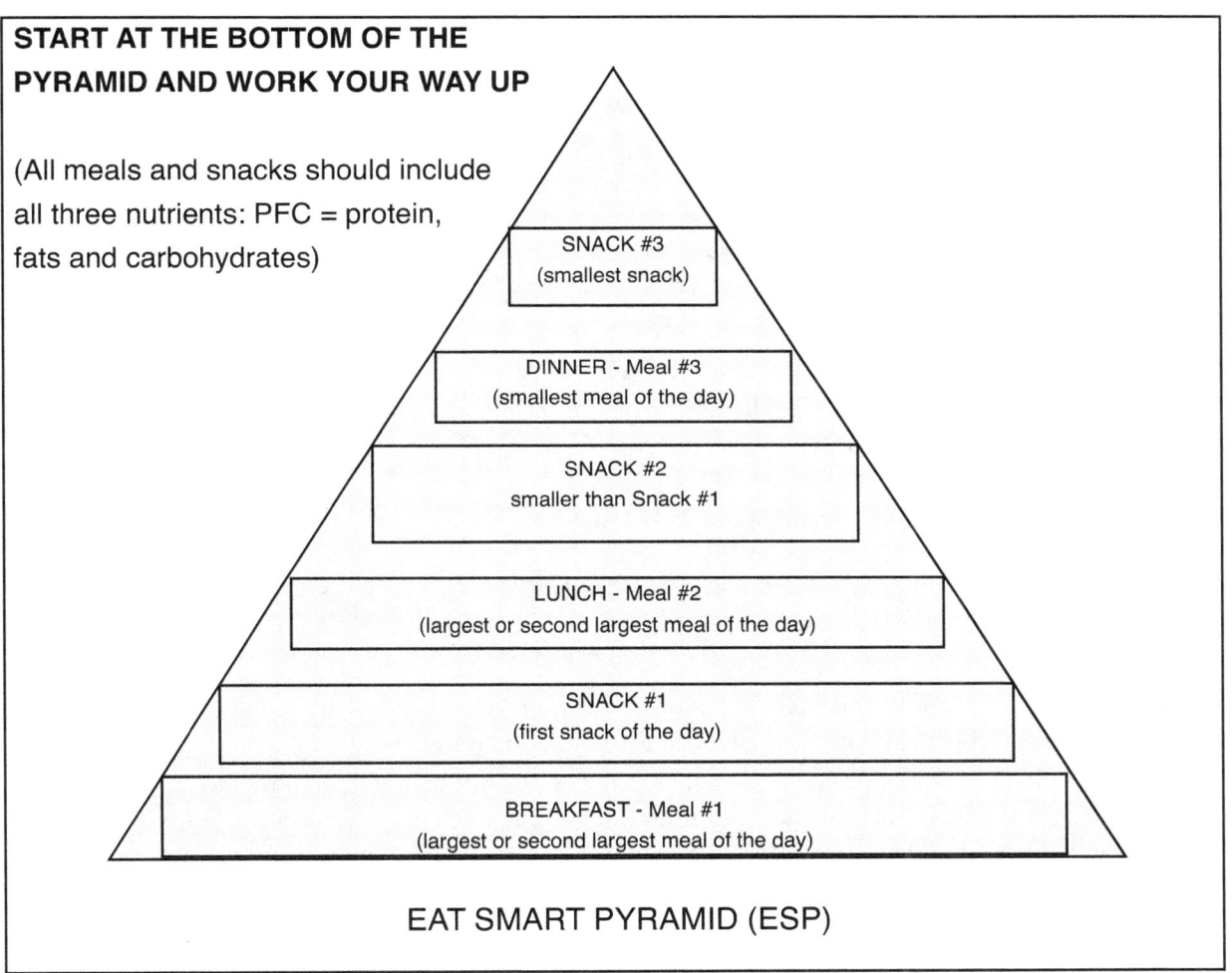

START AT THE BOTTOM OF THE PYRAMID AND WORK YOUR WAY UP

(All meals and snacks should include all three nutrients: PFC = protein, fats and carbohydrates)

SNACK #3
(smallest snack)

DINNER - Meal #3
(smallest meal of the day)

SNACK #2
smaller than Snack #1

LUNCH - Meal #2
(largest or second largest meal of the day)

SNACK #1
(first snack of the day)

BREAKFAST - Meal #1
(largest or second largest meal of the day)

EAT SMART PYRAMID (ESP)

GLYCEMIC INDEX (GI)

The glycemic index is a way of ranking carbohydrates. The scale scores carbohydrates from 1 to 100 based on the speed of energy release and the effect on blood sugar (glucose) levels. Foods with a low GI score *gradually* raise blood sugar levels. Foods with a high GI score *cause a sudden rise followed by a sudden drop* in blood sugar levels.

HIGH GI:

Foods with a GI greater than 70 are considered high on the scale. High GI carbs release energy rapidly causing a fast rise then a sudden crash in blood sugar (glucose) levels. *Eating high GI carbs can result in obesity.*

MODERATE GI:

Foods with a GI in the mid 50's up to 69 are deemed moderate and release energy at a moderate level.

LOW GI:

Foods with a GI less than 55 are considered low on the scale and slowly release energy causing a slow rise in blood sugar levels.

Why Should We Care About GI and What Is It Used For?

Knowing about the Glycemic Index is key to long-term health, reducing the risk of heart disease, diabetes and obesity.

1. Eat or drink high GI carbs or drinks for post workout <u>nutrition</u> when you need a boost of energy fast.
2. Eat or drink low GI carbs if you have blood sugar regulation problems.
3. It is best to try to eat or drink low GI carbs (slow releasing) as much as possible as they produce small changes in blood glucose and insulin levels. So much better for your body. Forcing your body to deal with high GI carbs on a routine basis can lead to type 2 diabetes, heart disease and obesity.
4. You can slow down the release of high GI foods by adding some protein or healthy fats. For example, a strawberry shake with added protein powder.

On the next page is a table with examples of high, medium and low GI carbs.

EXAMPLES OF HIGH, MEDIUM AND LOW GLYCEMIC INDEX CARBS

Low GI (1 - 55)		Med GI (56 - 69)		High GI (70 - 100)	
Peanuts	14	Boiled potato	56	White bread	71
Spinach	15	Mangoes	56	Millet	71
Cherries	22	Apricots	57	Watermelon	72
Bean sprouts	25	White pita bread	57	Microwave popcorn	72
Grapefruit	25	Instant oatmeal	58	Bagel	72
Low fat yogurt	33	White rice	58	Graham crackers	74
Apple	38	Cola	58	Potato chips	75
Apple juice	41	Danish pastry	59	Waffle	76
Spaghetti	42	Ice cream	61	Doughnut	76
Carrot juice	45	Hamburger bun	61	Weetabix	77
Carrot	47	Plain corn chips	63	Rice cakes	77
Oranges	48	Shortbread	64	Broad beans	79
Steel cut oats	49	Macaroni and cheese	64	Jelly beans	80
Whole grain bread	50	Raisins	64	Rice Krispies	82
Orange juice	52	Couscous	65	Cornflakes	83
Bananas	52	Pineapple	66	Pretzels	83
Sweet potato	54	Muesli (average)	66	Baked potato	85
Potato chips	54	Croissant	67	Brown rice pasta	92
Popcorn	55	Rye crisps	67	Baguette	95
Snickers Bar	55	Sugar (sucrose)	68	Fruit roll-ups	99
Brown rice	55	Orange soda	68	Glucose	100

STEP SEVEN - DIET REVIEW

QUICK FOOD TIPS

1. *SUGAR: AVOID IT LIKE THE PLAGUE*

- Avoid white processed sugar and by-products
- Sugar is the number one enemy for fat loss and good health
- Sugar releases insulin, a hormone that helps store excess calories as fat

2. *WATER: DRINK IT LIKE A CAMEL*

- Keep well hydrated; drink lots of water
- Drink about 8 to 12 glasses of water per day depending on your body size and activity level

3. *EAT LARGER PORTIONS EARLIER IN THE DAY*

- Eat for the coming event - more if you'll be very active and less if less active

4. *ALL CARBOHYDRATES ARE NOT EQUAL*

- Use the Glycemic Index as a guide (see the previous page for information) and www.glycemicindex.com. Eat slow-releasing carbohydrates
- Examples of good carbs - vegetables, sprouts, quinoa, rice, millet, spelt, sweet potatoes and some fruits
- Examples of bad carbs - processed foods, candy, soda and sugar
- You can slow down the release of high GI foods by adding some protein or healthy fats. For example, a strawberry shake with added protein powder.

5. *ALL FATS ARE NOT EQUAL*

- Examples of good fats - fish or flaxseed oil, avocado, olives, raw nuts, olive oil, whole eggs, coconut oil
- Your body needs good fats to increase metabolism
- Examples of bad fats - saturated (animal) fats, canola oil, margarine, fake butter, hydrogenated oils (found in many processed foods)

6. *ALL FOODS ARE NOT EQUAL*

- Real food or natural foods are much better for you than man-made manufactured foods with chemical additives
- Natural foods: vegetables, nuts, fruits, uncooked foods. Eat lots of natural foods
- Processed foods: contain lots of sugar, salt, preservatives, additives and harmful chemicals which affect your liver (the liver handles toxins in the body)
- Avoid artificial sweeteners, high fructose corn syrup and processed soy products

7. *FOCUS ON QUALITY OF FOOD RATHER THAN COUNTING CALORIES*

8. *CREATE A GOOD METABOLISM*

- Build muscle through strength training
- Eat nutritionally-dense natural foods

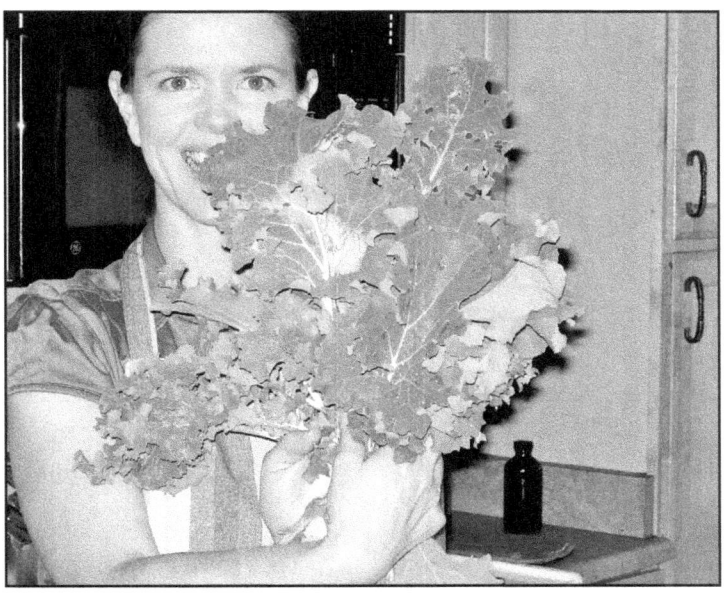

Kale is a great source of fiber, vitamins

and minerals

STEP EIGHT - TEST, MEASURE, RECORD

WHAT IS YOUR STARTING POINT?

It's very important to know what condition your body is in and what its capabilities are before you start your quest to improve your fitness, tone your muscles and lose weight. It's equally important to regularly check how you're doing as you go along.

Regular testing and body measurements will help you keep track of your progress. It will tell you if you're on track and going in the right direction or not. It will also take the guesswork out of what you are doing and make it scientific and objective so you have the right data on what actions to continue to do or what you need to change.

Once you have done some of the tests you will have an idea of what to improve and also have a way to keep track of your progress. Redo the tests every <u>4 to 8 weeks</u>, depending on how many workouts and diet changes you make along the way.

Keeping records is like having gauges on your car or an airplane. Would you fly an airplane with no flight gauges? Records are like gauges because they give you constant feedback. For fat loss, keeping a log or record of what you eat and your exercise minutes each day would be useful. Records keep you informed and in control because they let you know what to change or focus on precisely. The following tests will give you specific information about current strengths and weaknesses regarding different types of fitness that address different areas of your body.

SIMPLE FITNESS TESTS TO MEASURE AND RECORD YOUR PROGRESS

The following basic fitness tests and measurements will establish your starting strengths and weaknesses. This will let you know what to fix or improve and will help you select the level of difficulty you need to start from whether entry, intermediate or advanced.

You may find that you'll need to strengthen or stretch some weak or tight areas to improve and create a useful, functional and well-balanced body to further improve the quality of your daily life.

Testing and measuring will include measuring body size, circumference and fat levels as well as your aerobic fitness, flexibility and strength levels.

FIVE BASIC AREAS OF FITNESS YOU CAN TEST

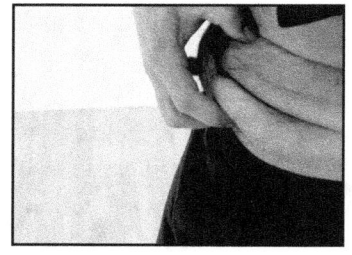

Fat test

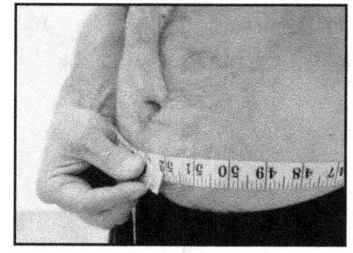

Girth / circumference

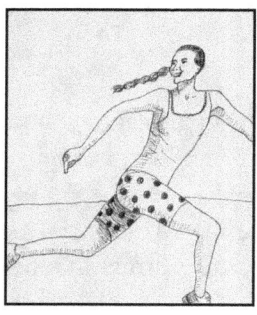

Cardio

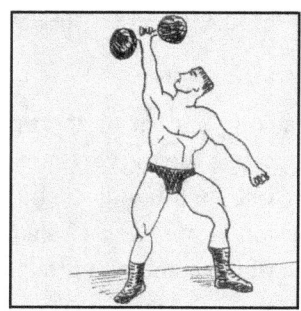

Strength

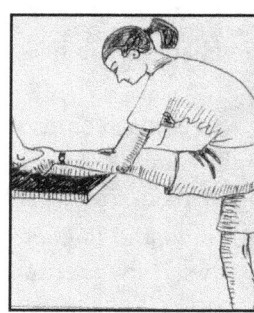

Flexibility

Some people think a person is fit and healthy if she doesn't look over or under weight and doesn't have a debilitating disease. She might look "normal" or in "proportion" when dressed in regular clothes but when you fat test her, you might find high fat levels. The skinny person may also have high body fat levels despite looking skinny or small; this is your "skinny fat" person.

Someone may look "healthy" or "normal" but can't bend down to touch her toes without difficulty, strain or possible injury. This person may not be able to jog for two minutes without gasping for air or experiencing some lower back or knee pain.

Defining health as disease-free is inadequate. Healthy should be more than disease-free; it should include functional strength, muscle tone, heart and lung fitness (aerobic/cardio fitness) and some flexibility. This would enable a person to meet the daily basic functions of living and recreation with some quality. Skiing, hiking or even a little rough-housing with your teenager should not hold much worry of possible injury.

STEP EIGHT - TEST MEASURE RECORD

IMPORTANT NOTE:

The following are simple low-tech methods to measure & record your fitness. Consult your physician before doing any fitness testing or measuring and before beginning or making changes to your diet or exercise program for diagnosis and treatment of illness and injuries. Do not make use of any of the information in this book unless you are in good health and received approval from your personal physician.

Let's briefly go over the five areas you can test. Each one will be covered in greater detail in the next pages so you'll know exactly how to do each test correctly.

- **GIRTH/CIRCUMFERENCE:** Circumference is a measurement you can do with a simple measuring tape to measure around your limbs and torso. If your waist (smallest part of torso) is larger than your hips (around the buttocks) it is indicative of being over-weight or obese.

- **BODY FAT:** High body fat levels have been associated with many health problems and even death. If your goal is weight or fat loss, concentrate on shrinking fat cells and preserving lean tissue (muscle) as a high priority.

- **CARDIO/AEROBIC FITNESS:** A simple way to test your aerobic fitness is to test your aerobic/anaerobic threshold - the point when your body switches from aerobic (oxygen) to an-aerobic (non-oxygen) sources of energy. This will be your current aerobic limit.

- **MUSCLE STRENGTH:** There are several methods of strength training, each yielding different results. One common method used in gyms is strength endurance training where you do high repetitions (more than 12 repetitions). This is good for muscle endurance, sports and everyday living. Another is muscle tone or hypertrophy (muscle building). This is more popular and where you do 6 to 12 repetitions to about 70, 80, 90 and occasionally 100% effort. This method will increase your strength, tone and build muscle and will in turn create a higher metabolic rate which is great for fat loss. Creating a strong body through a balanced program improves function and quality of life.

- **FLEXIBILITY:** Flexibility is the ability to bend, twist or turn in many different directions or planes of motion without stiffness, pain, strain or much discomfort. Being flexible also improves function and quality of life, especially for the aging adult.

TEST #1: BODY GIRTH
(CIRCUMFERENCE)

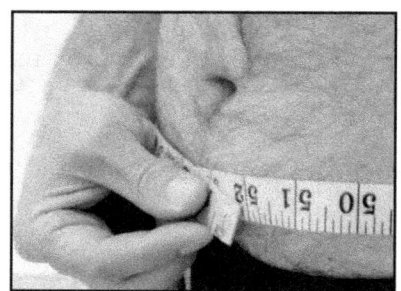

Measure the Distance Around Your Torso and Limbs

Our purpose here is to find out the starting size of your torso and limbs. Once you know this, you can re-measure every four weeks to find out whether there was a reduction in this measurement (or an increase if you're more interested in building muscle).

Follow the instructions below to get your current body girth measurements. On the next page is a form for recording your measurements, it also has tips for how to measure specific parts of the body.

- Get a standard tape measure (like the ones used in sewing kits).

- Use the tape measure to take the measurements recommended on the next page. Measure the right side of the body (if right-handed) or the left side (if left-handed). Take the average of three measurements and write that down in the Body Girth Measurements Form. Make sure you put today's date in the box above your measurement.

- Keep this chart updated every four weeks to monitor changes.

QUICK TIPS:

Measure your body from top to bottom: chest and back, upper arms, waist, around belly button, hips (for girls), thighs and calves. Get a friend or family member to help you if needed. Measure right side (or left if left-handed) three times, write down the average measurement. It's OK to measure both sides of the body, especially if you had a broken limb in the past. Make sure the tape is level around the area you are measuring and hold the tape with a light grip (without your finger between your body and the tape).

TEST #1: BODY GIRTH MEASUREMENTS FORM

CHEST AND BACK (around the chest and back, under arm pits)

WHEN TO MEASURE	TODAY	WEEK 4	WEEK 8	WEEK 12	WEEK 16	WEEK 20	WEEK 24
DATE							

Chest and Back (under armpits)							

QUICK TIPS FOR CHEST AND BACK: Measure mid-chest and make sure tape doesn't droop below shoulder blades at the back of your body. Gently breathe in and out. Take the average of 3 measurements.

UPPER ARMS (mid biceps and triceps. Use bent arm; relaxed)

Biceps and Triceps (mid-upper arm)							

QUICK TIPS FOR ARMS: Bend arm at 90 degree angle (as if showing off your muscles), measure largest part about mid-arm.

WAIST (smallest part of your torso)

Waist (smallest part of torso)							

QUICK TIPS FOR WAIST: Measure around the smallest part of your midsection (some waists are higher than others) when viewed from the front after exhaling.

ABS/BELLY BUTTON

Abs/Belly Button (around belly button)							

QUICK TIPS FOR ABS/BELLY BUTTON: Measure around your tummy at the belly button. Keep tape firm.

HIPS (for women)

HIPS (at widest point)							

QUICK TIPS FOR HIPS: Measure below hip bones, around mid-buttocks. Measure where the buttocks are maximally extended when viewed from the side.

THIGHS (upper leg - under the groin)

Thighs (upper thigh)							

QUICK TIPS FOR THIGHS: Measure around the top of thigh, the largest round part, just under buttocks.

TEST #2: BODY FAT

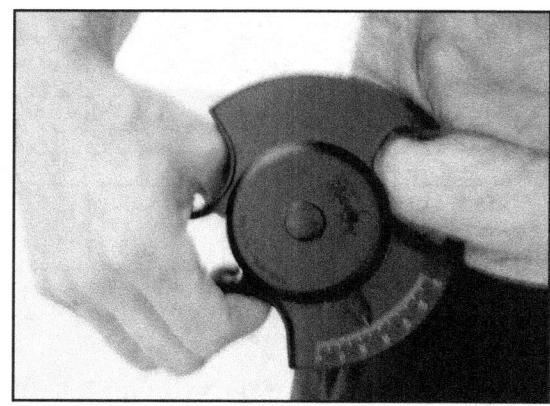

LOOKING GOOD HAS A LOT TO DO WITH HOW MUCH BODY FAT YOU HAVE

Body Composition: Fat Versus Lean Tissue

Body composition has everything to do with looking good in your skin. How lean or fat someone is has a lot to do with their body composition - the ratio of fat to lean tissue of the body.

Body composition can be simply defined as the amount of body fat tissue compared to lean tissue in your body.

Lean tissue is made up of muscle, bones, organs, blood, water and lymph.

Fat tissue is located in three main areas of the body. There are three basic types of fat:
VISCERAL FAT (found around organs): This is important to reduce for health reasons. You see this on large bellied men or women. Too much of this fat is dangerous to health.

INTRA-MUSCULAR FAT (found in muscles): Useful for aerobic athletes or people who do a lot of cardio exercise. Fat is stored in muscles and released for energy.

SUBCUTANEOUS FAT (found under the skin): This is what most people are trying to reduce to look leaner. This fat is what hides the shape of the muscles.

STEP EIGHT - TEST MEASURE RECORD

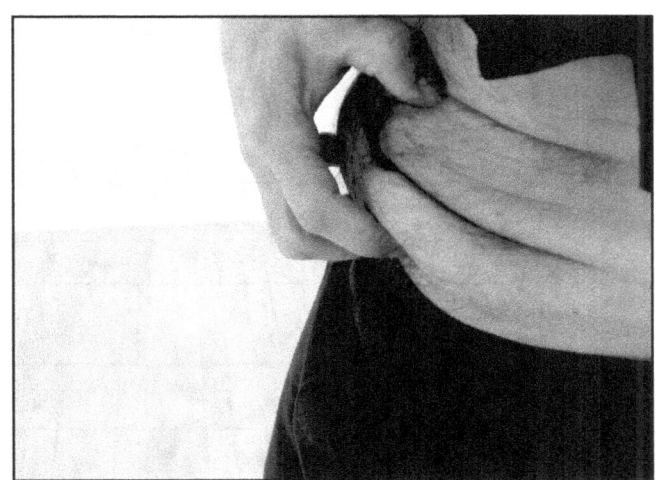

Now that you have a better understanding of the different kinds of fat in your body, you are going to get an idea of how much subcutaneous (under the skin) fat you have now. Once again, the purpose is to get a starting point so that as you go along you can re-measure and compare the results every four weeks to check on your progress.

Ideally you would use skin fold calipers but a simple ruler will do the job as well. To do this test, lightly pinch the skin with your thumb and index finger on the spot specified in the "Body Fat Measurement Form" on the next page, then measure the distance between your thumb and forefinger with your ruler. You can measure in either inches or millimeters (millimeters are more accurate). Measure the spot three times and take the average to record in the correct place on the "Body Fat Measurement Form" on the next page.

The form will guide you with tips on how to measure correctly. Don't forget to record today's date in the correct place so you know when you started. And don't worry, these measurements will change!

TEST #2: BODY FAT MEASUREMENT FORM

Measure each site three times and write down the average. Record results in inches or millimeters. *If you don't have fat calipers use a ruler instead as described on page 89.*

WHEN TO MEASURE	Today	Week 4	Week 8	Week 12	Week 16	Week 20	Week 24
DATE							

Biceps (mid point)							

QUICK TIP FOR BICEPS: Measure the middle part of the biceps muscle (front upper arm)

Triceps (mid point)							

QUICK TIP FOR TRICEPS: Measure middle part of triceps muscle (back of arm)

Rear Shoulder Blade (back of body)							

QUICK TIP FOR SHOULDER BLADE: Measure underneath the middle low part of the scapular blade (back of right shoulder blade)

Side of Hip (2 inches above)							

QUICK TIP FOR SIDE OF HIPS: Measure above the hip bone to the side (2 inches above right hip bone)

Belly Area (1 inch to right of belly button)							

QUICK TIP FOR BELLY: Measure to the right of the belly button (1 inch from the belly button)

Upper Thigh (Front and mid thigh)							

QUICK TIPS FOR THIGH: Measure the middle of the thigh at the front

Total in. or mm. (Add all measurements here)							

TEST #3: AEROBIC/CARDIO TEST
What is Your Anaerobic Threshold?

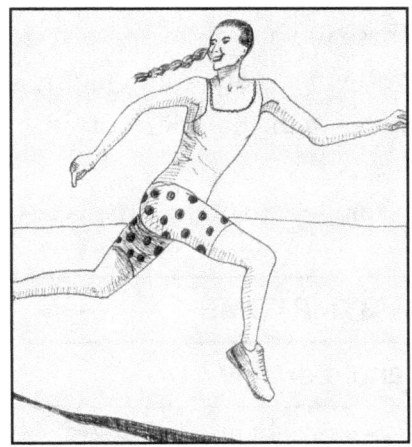

Small framed or small boned individuals are well suited to long distance running.

First, let's start with some definitions of words that get used very regularly when people talk about fitness:

- *Aerobic energy system* is when the body uses oxygen as its main source for fuel or energy.
- *Cardio is short for cardiovascular* which means heart and veins. Cardio exercises strengthen the heart and increase the effectiveness of the lungs. They can get you out of breath.
- *Anaerobic energy system* is when the body no longer uses oxygen as its main source of fuel or energy but instead taps into fuel reserves in the muscles.
- *Anaerobic threshold* is the point at which you switch from the aerobic energy system (using oxygen mainly) to the anaerobic energy system (using glycogen/carbohydrates stored in the muscles as the main source of energy or fuel).

The purpose of this test is to find out what your aerobic limit is (or your anaerobic threshold, to be more scientific). The fitter you are, the longer it will take before you start using your anaerobic energy system. Here is where you find out your starting point to compare your progress with every four to eight weeks.

AEROBIC TO ANAEROBIC STAGES

Over the years I have observed definite stages people go through as they increase their exercise intensity. You will notice these too as you increase your fitness levels. Basically they are the observable signals that tell you when you're moving from aerobic training (burning oxygen) to anaerobic (burning fuel stores in the muscles instead).

Below are these stages going from low to higher intensity - don't ever go past Stage 6.

STAGES	OBSERVATIONS/SYMPTOMS
1	Breathing easily and regularly
2	Breathing rate increases a little
3	Talk test: struggling a little to talk comfortably during activity
4	Starting to breathe a little hard
5	**Out of breath. You start to breathe a lot harder (breathing through mouth, mouth opens wide, deep breathing). You've hit your ANAEROBIC THRESHOLD**
6	Feel a little light headed - dizzy
7	Feel a little nauseous
8	Feel more than a little nauseous
9	Possibly vomit if you insist on pushing past this point
10	Pass out, faint (body goes horizontal)

If you are in good physical condition and have been approved by your physician to exercise you can push yourself to reach **Stage 5**: Out of breath (breathing hard). Otherwise go to **Stage 3**: Struggling to talk comfortably during activity only.

AEROBIC TO ANAEROBIC STAGES GRAPH

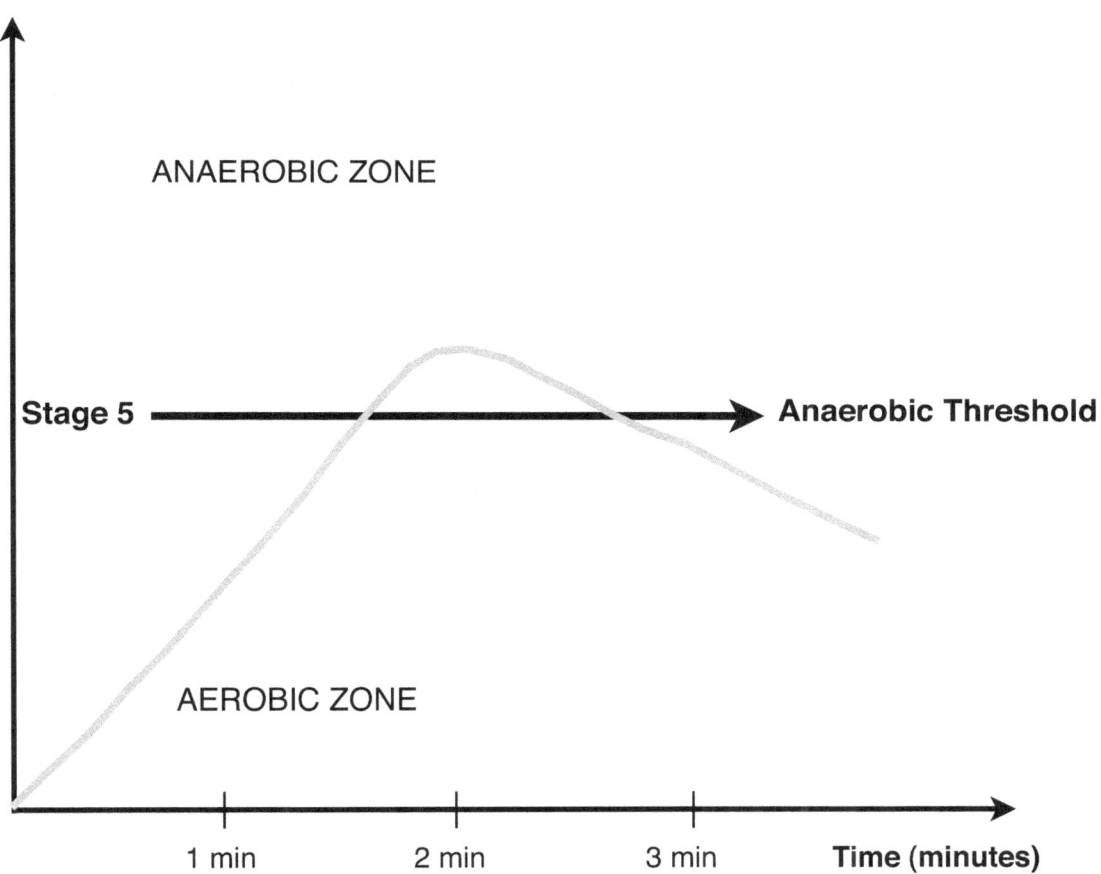

Usually if someone is slightly de-conditioned, the muscles that they are using to do the aerobic/cardio exercise will tire out or fatigue before they can get their heart rate up high enough to challenge the heart and lungs to get to the anaerobic threshold.

The body can only operate for up to 2 minutes in the anaerobic zone. Examples of anaerobic activities include 100m sprints, 400 to 800m dash, weight-lifting, fast or short-distance hill runs.

A simple way of interpreting the "Aerobic to Anaerobic Stages Graph" is to imagine how it would relate to a real person exercising. Let's use a man running as an example. Using the graph, we can see that it would take this man one and a half minutes of running to reach his anaerobic threshold. At this point he would be breathing hard through his mouth and unable to talk to you. He could continue in this state for about a minute and then would have to slow it down and return to his aerobic zone.

Moving into the anaerobic zone for short bursts of exercise is used in interval training, an increasingly popular method for increasing cardio fitness levels. With interval training you go from aerobic to anaerobic and back down to the aerobic zone. In other words, easy exercise to hard then back to easy. Per our table, "Aerobic to Anaerobic Stages" on page 92, a person doing interval training would be going from a Stage One to Stage Five, then back to a Stage Two for a bit then up to a Stage Five again and so on.

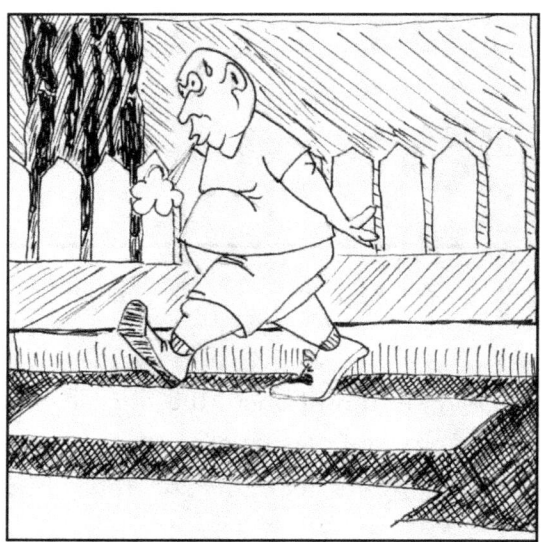

The more unfit you are, the faster you reach your
anaerobic threshold (Stage 5 - out of breath). Don't
quit, your body can get fit with regular aerobic activity.

AEROBIC/CARDIO TESTS

1.Resting Heart Rate Test:

Ideally take your heart rate first thing in the morning upon waking and after a good night's sleep. Otherwise take it before you do your aerobic test. Your resting heart rate get lower as you get fitter.

How to take Your Resting Heart Rate:
- •Use your first two fingers and gently press to feel a pulse on the left or right side of your throat or at your opposite inner wrist (under your thumb).
- •Use a clock or watch to count each pulse over a 15 second period.
- •Multiply the number of pulses counted over 15 seconds by 4 which will give you how many beats in 60 seconds. That is your resting heart rate per minute (or beats per minute - BPM).
- •Record the beats per minute on the form below.

QUICK TIPS:

Avoid using the thumb as it has a pulse of its own. Avoid pressing too hard on your pulse. Make sure you do this first thing in the morning.

RESTING HEART RATE TEST RESULTS

WHEN TO MEASURE	Today	Week 4	Week 8	Week 12	Week 16	Week 20	Week 24
DATE							
Resting Heart Rate at 15 seconds x 4 =							

QUICK TIP: No caffeine or alcohol 24 hours before this test. Count heart beats for 15 seconds and multiply by 4

2. The Walk, Jog or Run Test:

Three tests for three levels of fitness. Go to a park, field or other soft surface to do a walk, jog or run test and see how far and how long you can do it without stopping. You'll use this to compare your progress every four to eight weeks.

Entry Level (Walk/Jog) Test:
- •Walk (or jog if you can) until you start breathing hard and getting out of breath (reaching your anaerobic threshold). Time yourself from the start until you feel you have to stop.
- •Record the time and distance of this walk (or jog) on the "Entry and Intermediate Level Aerobic Test" form on the next page (use the stop watch tool on your cell phone for timing and count the number of laps you did for distance - try to do your future tests at the same location).

STEP EIGHT - TEST MEASURE RECORD

Intermediate Level Test:

- •Jog as far and for as long as you can. Time yourself.
- •Record the time and distance of this jog (or run) on the "Entry and Intermediate Level Aerobic Test" form below (use the stop watch tool on your cell phone for timing and count the number of laps you did for distance - try to do your future tests at the same location).

Don't worry if it was less than 3 minutes or even 30 seconds, all you want is a starting point for reference so you can compare later as you improve. If you experience any joint or muscle ache or pain, stop and record that fact.

ENTRY AND INTERMEDIATE LEVEL AEROBIC TEST

WHEN TO MEASURE	Today	Week 4	Week 8	Week 12	Week 16	Week 20	Week 24
DATE							
Walk or jog. How many minutes?							
Walk or jog. How many laps/distance?							
Heart rate immediately after test (check for 15 seconds x 4)							

QUICK TIP: Walk 3 minutes to warm up before jogging or running.

Advanced Level Testing:

If you are already quite fit try something more challenging like rope skipping, jump burpees or 3/4 pace sprints.

- •Choose one of the activities listed above and go as long as possible without stopping.
- •Time the duration or number of repetitions or both depending on the activity you choose. Record this data on the "Advanced Level Aerobic Test" form below.

ADVANCED LEVEL AEROBIC TEST

WHEN TO MEASURE	Today	Week 4	Week 8	Week 12	Week 16	Week 20	Week 24
DATE							
Rope skip, 3/4/sprint or burpees How many minutes/ repetitions?							
Heart rate immediately after test (check for 15 seconds x 4)							

TEST #4: STRENGTH TESTING
Major Muscle Groups

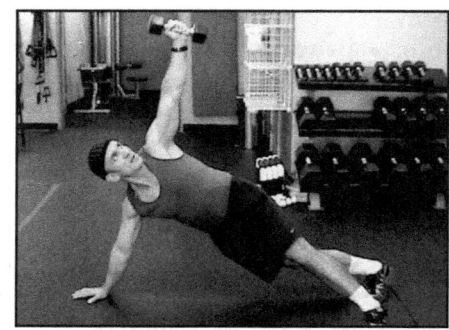

The purpose of Test #4 is to find out what your current strength levels are for major muscle groups in your body so that when you retest them later for comparison you can see what progress and improvement you have made. It will also help you to choose an exercise starting point based on your strengths and weaknesses, whether it be entry, intermediate or advanced level. Remember, your muscles hold you up, keep your back aligned, help with circulation and ensure you look fabulous (among many other things), so it's well-worth investing time to find out your strength starting point.

HOW TO DO STRENGTH TESTS
The 60 Second Muscular Strength Endurance Test

On the following pages you will find photos of the test exercises you will do in this section along with specific instructions for each.

There are three levels for each test: entry, intermediate and advanced.
Entry Level is the easiest level and is for anyone who is unfit or out of condition;
Intermediate Level is for those individuals who are of average fitness and strength levels. These people are usually active, playing some sport or going to the gym or doing a similar activity;
Advanced Level exercises or tests are for those who are already quite fit and in condition because of regular gym or sports activities. This is the most difficult level of testing and exercises.

It's very important, no matter what level you do, to do all exercises with *good exercise form*. If you can't continue the exercise with good form then immediately stop, despite being able to push through and do a few more. It's also important to select the right testing level for yourself (too easy and there will be no challenge; too hard and you won't be able to do the test with good exercise form and you may run the risk of some injury).

STEP EIGHT - TEST MEASURE RECORD

1. Do each exercise with good form, without stopping, for a total of 60 seconds. Don't worry if you can't go the distance. Just record the time and how many movements or repetitions you were able to do without stopping. This is your starting point.

2. Do not hold your breath during exercises and stop if you cannot continue to use good exercise form or if you feel any joint or nerve pain or discomfort.

3. Always start at a level you can do fairly easily. If you're new to exercise, Entry Level will be where you'd start. Experienced exercisers will likely choose intermediate or advanced level exercises.

4. If you are not sure of your current strength level start at the easiest level, Entry Level. If that is too easy and you can do it with good exercise form then move up to the next level.

As you do your fitness program on a regular basis you will notice increases in your energy, fitness and strength. You will be able to go to the next level of exercise difficulty.

On the next few pages you will find photos of the test exercises that you will do. Advanced Level being for the already conditioned person and the toughest, Intermediate is next and Entry is for the new person and is the easiest level. Start with the easiest level and work your way up to the tougher levels. Do all exercises with *good exercise form*. It is important to select the right testing level.

There is a form for recording your strength testing results on page 105.

TEST LEG STRENGTH: THE SQUAT

Target Area: Thighs and Buttocks

Record the number of squats you can do correctly in 60 seconds on page 109. The squats must be done in the form explained and illustrated below.

Hands Out Front Squats

Overhead Ball Squats

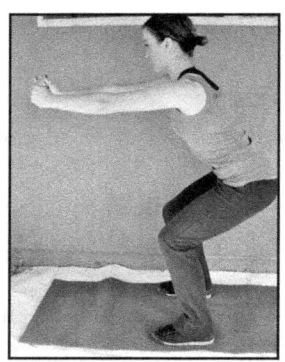

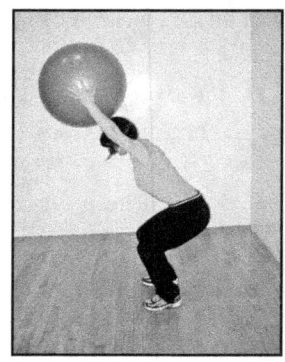

Entry or Intermediate

Advanced

1. Stand with feet pointed straight ahead and hip/shoulder width apart

2. Keep knees behind your toes as you squat

3. Keep your bottom & hips slightly sticking out (keeps your spine lightly arched)

4. Squat until your bottom is slightly higher than your knees (thighs are not quite parallel to the floor)

5. Stand up until knees are 95% straight/almost straight – do not lock your knees. Repeat for 60 seconds

6. RECORD YOUR RESULTS IN THE STRENGTH TESTS RECORD FORM ON PAGE 105

SAFETY TIPS:
- **Do not hold your breath during any of the exercises**
- **Do not lock or over-bend any joints**
- **Stop any time you want to or if you experience any joint pain**

TEST CHEST STRENGTH: THE PUSH-UP

Target area: Chest, Front Shoulders, Back of Upper Arm

Record how many push-ups you can do with good exercise form in 60 seconds. The push-ups must be done in the form explained and illustrated below.

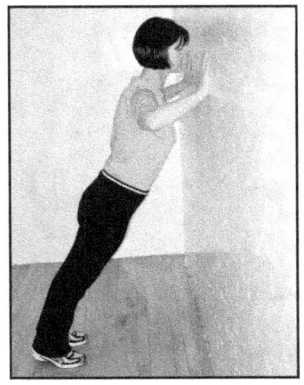

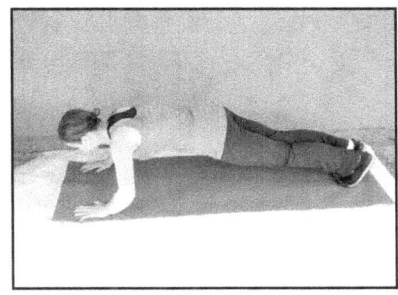

Entry Level
Wall Push-up

Intermediate Level
Knee Push-up

Advanced Level
Full Push-up

ENTRY LEVEL: Stand with feet pointed straight ahead and hip/shoulder width apart about 2 feet from the wall.

INTERMEDIATE LEVEL: Place knees on floor, feet and knees shoulder width apart.

ADVANCED LEVEL: Place feet shoulder width apart, hands under shoulders .

1. Start with your arms about 95% straight, then lower your body while keeping your torso straight

2. Return to start position and repeat for the next 60 seconds

3. RECORD YOUR RESULTS IN THE STRENGTH TESTS RECORD FORM ON PAGE 105

SAFETY TIPS:
- **Do not hold your breath during any of the exercises. Take one breath per movement or repetition**
- **Do not lock or over-bend any joints and stop at any point you want or if you experience any joint or nerve pain**
- **Keep your back straight. If your back sags or you feel pressure there, stop**

TEST BACK AND ARM STRENGTH: THE PULL-UP
Target area: Back, Rear Shoulders, Front of Upper Arm

Record how many pull-ups you can do with good form in 60 seconds. The pull-ups must be done in the form explained and illustrated below.

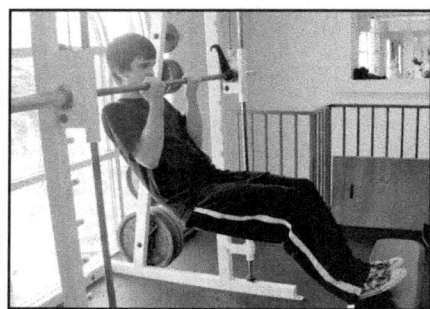

Entry or Intermediate Level

Horizontal Chins

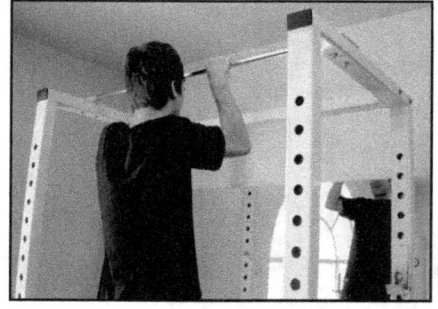

Advanced level

Vertical Chins

ENTRY LEVEL: Hold the bar with overhand grip slightly wider than shoulders with while hanging with bottom off the ground and heels resting on a bench (knees slightly bent).

INTERMEDIATE LEVEL: Hold the bar with overhand grip slightly wider than shoulders with while hanging with bottom off the ground and heels resting on a bench (knees slightly bent).

ADVANCED LEVEL: Hold the bar with overhand grip slightly wider than shoulders with feet pointed straight ahead and hip/shoulder width apart.

1. Start with your arms 95% straight (elbow joint not locked or fully straightened) and raise your body – keep torso straight, repeat for the next 60 seconds. Intermediate and Advanced only (**Entry Level** will just hold onto the bar with arms 90% bent and chin near the bar for 60 seconds, or as long as possible if 60 seconds is too long)

2. RECORD YOUR RESULTS IN THE STRENGTH TESTS RECORD FORM ON PAGE 105

SAFETY TIPS:
• **Do not hold your breath with any of the exercise**
• **Do not lock or over-bend any joints**
• **Stop any time you want to or if you experience any joint pain**

TEST CORE AND ABDOMINAL STRENGTH: THE SIT-UP OR CRUNCH
Target area: Rectus Abdominus (front abs)

Record the number of sit-ups or crunches done correctly in 60 seconds. The sit-ups or crunches must be done in the form explained and illustrated.

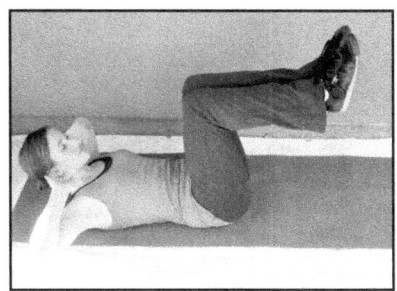

Entry or Intermediate Level

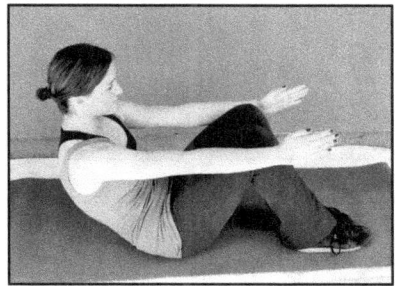

Intermediate (feet anchored)

Advanced (feet not anchored)

ENTRY LEVEL:

1. Crunches. See instructions for Intermediate Level (below) on how to do crunches.

INTERMEDIATE LEVEL (CRUNCHES OR SIT-UPS):

1. Two choices. One is to do crunches, the other is the same as the Advanced Level but your feet are anchored under a bed/couch or someone is holding them down
2. For crunches, lie on floor with feet up in the air or resting on a chair with knees at 90 degrees and hands by the ears. Lift shoulders off the ground and bring your chest towards your navel. Do not pull at your head or neck
3. Keep elbows out/apart and return to start position. Repeat for 60 seconds

ADVANCED LEVEL:

1. Lie on the floor with feet hip to shoulder-width apart, pointing straight ahead and not anchored. Knees 90% bent, hands on thighs. Slowly lift shoulders off the ground
2. Start by sitting up until your elbows are in line with your knees at the top of the sit-up
3. Return to start position and repeat for 60 seconds

RECORD YOUR RESULTS IN THE STRENGTH TESTS RECORD FORM ON PAGE 105

SAFETY TIPS:

- **Do not hold your breath, lock or over-bend joints**
- **Stop anytime you want to or if you experience any joint pain**
- **Keep your back rounded. If your back arches or you feel pressure in the lower back area, stop**

TEST CONDITIONING: THE BURPEE

Target area: Full Body Strength and Conditioning

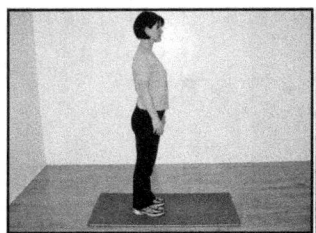 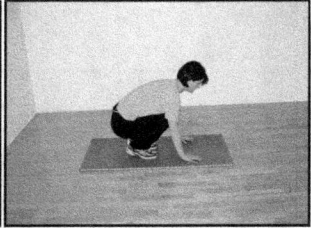 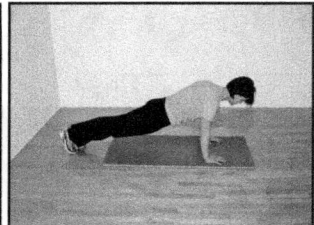 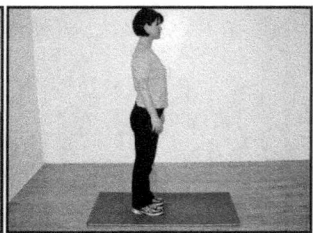

Start	Walk or jump your feet out	Finish

ENTRY AND INTERMEDIATE LEVELS: You will walk out and then stand up at the end. No explosive movements.

ADVANCED LEVEL: You will jump out and then up at the finish. Explosive movements.

1. Stand with feet pointed straight ahead, hip or shoulder-width apart

2. Keep knees 95% straight; don't fully lock or straighten your knees

3. Keep your lower back/spine lightly arched and knees behind toes as you squat

4. Squat until your hands touch the ground. Walk (Entry or Intermediate) or jump (Advanced) your feet back until you are in a push-up position

5. Walk (Entry or Intermediate) or jump (Advanced) your feet back under your thighs. Stand (Entry or Intermediate) or jump (Advanced) up to start position

6. Repeat for a duration of 60 seconds

RECORD YOUR RESULTS IN THE STRENGTH TESTS RECORD FORM ON PAGE 105

STRENGTH TESTS RECORD FORM

Use the form below when you test and retest yourself to record your strength testing information every 4 weeks.

STRENGTH TESTS RECORD FORM

STRENGTH TESTS (60 seconds max)	Date:	Date:	Date:	Date:	Date:	Date:	Date:
TEST 1. Squats							
TEST 2. Push-ups (full, knee or wall)							
TEST 3. Chins/Pull-ups (vertical or horizontal)							
TEST 4. Sit-ups or Crunches							
TEST 5. Burpees: Advanced, Intermediate or Entry							
TEST 6. Any other you want to add							

QUICK TIP: Don't worry if you lasted less than 60 seconds or even 30 seconds. This is a starting point. Remember, if you experience any joint or muscle ache or pain, stop and record that on the form.

TEST #5: FLEXIBILITY - THE SIT AND REACH
Back of Legs and Back

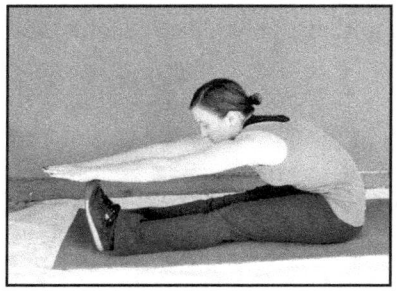

The Sit and Reach Test

You can do a simple and general flexibility test, the Sit and Reach. This will give you an idea of the flexibility you have in two basic areas: the lower back and rear of the legs (also known as the hamstrings).

Gently stretch forward only once, without practicing the stretch or warming up the muscles. You want to see your flexibility as it would be in everyday life. Stretch forward only to the point of slight discomfort, not pain, and hold the stretch for 5 to 10 seconds while you record the distance from your hands to your toes. Your hands will end up either in front of or behind your toes.

All you want is a starting point to compare future tests to see improvements as you include stretches in your overall balanced workout program.

1. Start the Sit-and-Reach stretch by sitting upright on the floor (legs 99% straight)
2. Both legs are straight out in front, keep your back straight without bending the top half of your back. Keep your chest out and shoulders pulled back and down
3. Slowly lean forward from the hips (keep your back straight), sliding both hands as far forward down your shins as possible (to slight discomfort, not pain) and hold
4. Record the distance from fingertips to toes on the Flexibility Test Record Form on the next page

QUICK TIP:
Avoid bouncing at the end of the stretch (called ballistic stretching). This can cause micro tears in the muscles or tendons creating scar tissue which then makes you tighter than before.

FLEXIBILITY TEST RECORD FORM

	Today	Week 4	Week 8	Week 12	Week 16	Week 20	Week 24
FLEXIBILITY TEST	Date:	Date:	Date:	Date:	Date:	Date:	Date:
Sit and Reach (in in. or cm)							

QUICK TIP: If you have any injuries that may be affected by doing this stretch, do not do it. Bend form the hips, not the mid to upper back. Keep your lower back in its natural curve.

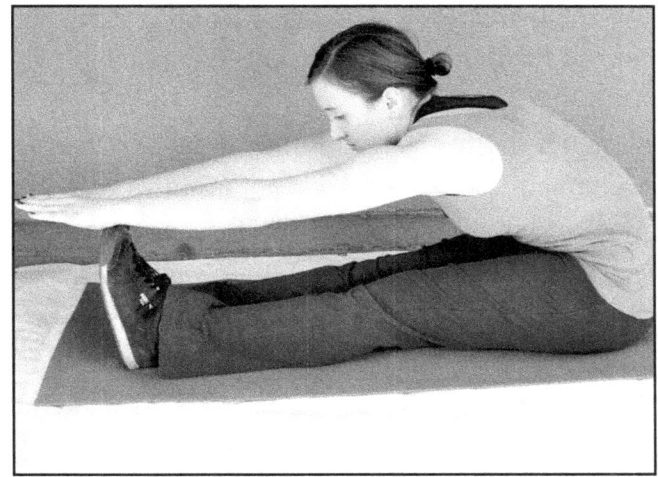

Sit & Reach test: If your hands go in front of your feet while you maintain a straight back, the number recorded is in the positive range. Anything behind your toe is negative. Example: fingers go past toes comfortably = plus 2 inches. Behind toes by 2 inches will be referred to as negative 2 inches.

EXERCISE TRACKING FORMS

It's very important to keep a record of your daily and weekly progress once you start exercising. Periodic testing, measuring and recording will take the guesswork out of what you are doing and will objectively inform you as to whether what you are doing is successful or not.

I have included three tracking and recording forms (two four-week short forms and one sixteen-week long form) for you to fill out and use each day. I have also included a filled-out sample form to demonstrate how to use the forms.

These forms will help you:
- Set and track goals for the first four to sixteen weeks
- Track the number of workouts done per day or week
- Track the number of exercise minutes done per day or week
- Track your total body weight and fat to lean tissue ratio
- Track strength, cardio and flexibility improvements and plateaus

There are three sections on the forms - body fat %, fat lbs, lean lbs - for which you will need a scale that gives weight and fat percentages. Some scales will give you your lean and fat weights as well, but if not, multiply your weight by the percentage of fat given on the scale; this will give your weight in fat. Take this and subtract it from your total weight to find your lean weight.

For example, if you weigh 150 pounds and have 25% body fat, you then multiply 150 by 25% to get 37.5 pounds of fat. You would subtract 37.5 from 150 to get 112.5 pounds which is your lean weight.

If you don't have a way to work out your body fat percentage, then leave the three sections (start body fat %, fat lbs and lean lbs) blank for now.

On the next page you can see the sample "Four-Week Activity Form" filled out for Mrs. I M N Action. The idea is that you discover how these forms can be used to help you track your own progress to achieve your goals. Following the sample you'll find the blank forms for your own use.

Rudi M Personal Training Systems
Four-Week Activity Form

YOUR NAME: *Mrs I M N Action*	DATE STARTED: *January 10, 2011*

Start weight: *200lb*	Start body fat %: *30%*	Fat weight: *60lb*	Lean weight: *140lb*
Long term goal weight: *140lb*	Long term goal, body fat: *20%*	Long term goal, fat weight: *28lb*	Long term goal, lean weight: *112lb*

Week + date	Mon min	Tue min	Wed min	Thu min	Fri min	Sat min	Sun min	Total Minutes	Weight in lbs	Fat %	Fat lb	Lean lb
1. *Jan 10 to 17, 2011*	20	0	20	0	20	0	0	60 min	200	30	60	140
2. *Jan 18 to 25, 2011*	30	20	20	30	20	0	0	120 min	199.5	29.8	59.45	140.04
3. *Jan 26 to Feb 2, 2011*	30	20	20	30	20	0	0	120 min	198	29	57.42	140.58
4. *Feb 3 to 10, 2011*	60	20	60	30	20	30	0	220 min	196	28.5	55.86	140.14

Progress comments: *It is getting easier as I am getting into a rhythm. I started to feel good after the first 2 weeks. I've dropped 4 lbs of fat (1 per week). I would like to lose more but I know the body can only lose 1 to 2 pounds a week per the ACSM* so I can't complain and I am not losing any muscle, which is great.*

From this sample form you can see that total body weight, body fat percentage and body fat weight are all decreasing while lean weight is stable and slightly up (healthy). The most successful day was Wednesday and Week 4 was the most successful week with 220 exercise minutes done.

Copy and use the forms on the next pages to keep track of your activities.

*ACSM: American College of Sports Medicine (gold standard in fitness certification)

Rudi M Personal Training Systems
First Four-Week Activity Form

YOUR NAME:	DATE STARTED:

Start weight:	Start body fat %:	Start fat weight:	Start lean weight:
Long term goal weight:	Long term goal, body fat %:	Long term goal, fat weight:	Long term goal, lean weight:

Week + date	Mon min	Tue min	Wed min	Thu min	Fri min	Sat min	Sun min	Total Minutes	Weight in lbs	Fat %	Fat lb	Lean lb
1												
2												
3												
4												

Progress comments:

8 Simple Steps

STEP EIGHT - TEST MEASURE RECORD

Rudi M Personal Training Systems
Second Four-Week Activity Form

YOUR NAME:		DATE STARTED:	

Start weight:	Start body fat %:	Start fat weight:	Start lean weight:
Long term goal weight:	Long term goal, body fat %:	Long term goal, fat weight:	Long term goal, lean weight:

Week + date	Mon min	Tue min	Wed min	Thu min	Fri min	Sat min	Sun min	Total Minutes	Weight in lbs	Fat %	Fat lb	Lean lb
1												
2												
3												
4												

Progress comments:

Rudi M Personal Training Systems
Sixteen-Week Activity Form

YOUR NAME:						DATE STARTED:						

Start weight:				Start body fat %:				Start fat weight:			Start lean weight:	
Long term goal weight:				Long term goal, body fat %:				Long term goal, fat weight:			Long term goal, lean weight:	

Week + date	Mon min	Tue min	Wed min	Thu min	Fri min	Sat min	Sun min	Total Minutes	Weight in lbs	Fat %	Fat lb	Lean lb
1												
2												
3												
4												
5												
6												
7												
8												
9												
10												
11												
13												
14												
15												
16												

Progress comments:

EXERCISE SAFETY TIPS

EXERCISE SAFETY TIPS

How to Achieve Maximal Exercise Safety, Form and Results

- Do not over-bend (flex) a joint

- Do not straighten or lock a joint (hyper extension)

- Do not bounce at the end of a stretch (ballistic stretching)

- Do warm up, stretch, work out, cool down and stretch with all workouts

- Learn and apply perfect exercise form

- Learn and apply the seven posture checkpoints to all exercises and physical activities (see page 118)

- Learn and apply the 8 Golden Rules of Exercise and Fitness (see page 119)

- Balance your workouts. Include all three basics: strength, stretch and cardio exercises

- To improve any area of fitness you must gradually challenge yourself when you exercise

- Breathe. Avoid holding your breath when exercising

PERFECT EXERCISE FORM

There is an ideal way to align your body and posture no matter whether you are at rest, moving, at work or doing a challenging activity, workout or sport.

If someone is sedentary for long periods or many years and also has a body that is misaligned (has poor posture), this will create weaknesses, imbalances and gradual wear and tear on muscles, tendons, ligaments or joints. If a person is very active and has poor posture or body alignment, the wear and tear will accelerate at a fast rate.

How do you tell if your posture and joints are in correct alignment when sedentary or active?

There are several key areas to align, starting with your feet, knees, lower back and hips, shoulders, head and neck, elbows and wrists. The idea is to keep these parts in what's called "neutral position", so that stress and strain to muscles, tendons, ligaments, joints, the spine or nerves is reduced. This is the ideal position for your body to be in. The area is not over-flexed (bent) or over-extended (arched) or over-rotated internally or externally. Neutral position helps keep your total body or body segment in the ideal and proper alignment or posture.

Some tools or ways to get feedback on your posture:

- use a large wall mirror

- use a video camera to video your body in motion

- find someone to check on your key posture points

Focus on perfect exercise form and technique when exercising. Stop if your form is lost for any reason. Work targeted areas. If the targeted area tires and another area does the work, stop and rest.

There are 7 posture checkpoints that actually undercut any and all basic movements or exercise. These are the foundations for all good exercise form and technique. Knowing them and using them will help maximize safety and results.

The 7 Posture Checkpoints
For Maximum Safety and Results

Checkpoint 1: FEET (applies to nearly all exercises)
- FRONT VIEW: Feet pointed straight ahead and shoulder to hip-width apart
- REAR VIEW: Feet pointed straight ahead

Checkpoint 2: KNEES (applies to nearly all standing exercises)
- FRONT VIEW: Knees pointed straight ahead, hip to shoulder-width apart
- SIDE VIEW: Knees slightly bent when standing. When squatting, knees kept behind toes
- REAR VIEW: Knees pointed straight ahead, not turned in or out

Checkpoint 3: LOWER BACK/PELVIS (applies to exercises that involve bending and squats)
- REAR VIEW: Top of both hips parallel to the ground, no tilt
- SIDE VIEW: Lower back in neutral position, spine slightly arched (natural curve)
- FRONT VIEW: Top of both hips parallel to the ground, no tilt

Checkpoint 4: SHOULDERS (applies to nearly all exercises)
- FRONT VIEW: Shoulders parallel to the ground, no tilt
- SIDE VIEW: Chest out, shoulders pulled back and down
- REAR VIEW: Shoulders parallel to the ground, no tilt

Checkpoint 5: NECK/HEAD (applies to exercises that involve bending and squats)
- SIDE VIEW: Neck in neutral position, natural curve of the neck
- FRONT VIEW: Look straight ahead, no head rotation or tilt to the side
- REAR VIEW: Look straight ahead, no head rotation or tilt to the side

Checkpoint 6: ELBOWS (applies to some exercises)
- For the majority of exercises, keep elbows in line with your shoulders and wrists. Example, biceps curl, chin-ups or lat pull-downs

Checkpoint 7: WRISTS (applies to some exercises)
- For the majority of exercises, keep wrists straight and in line with the forearms. Example, biceps curl, chin-ups or lat pull-downs.

EXERCISE SAFETY TIPS

8 Golden Rules of Exercise and Fitness

1. BREATHE
- Don't hold breath
- Don't breathe too shallowly or too deeply
- Mostly breathe out on exertion

2. CHOOSE THE RIGHT ACTIVITY
- Choose the activity that will lead to or can get you to your goals
- To get stronger, apply progressive overload when you do resistance or strength training
- To increase flexibility, stretch to the point of slight discomfort
- To improve heart and lung fitness, do aerobic or cardio exercises until you get out of breath, several times

3. PERFORM PERFECT EXERCISE FORM AND TECHNIQUE
- Once you have chosen the right exercise to help you achieve your goals:
- DO THE EXERCISE CORRECTLY BY USING THE 7 CHECKPOINTS
- VERIFY THAT YOUR EXERCISE FORM IS CORRECT BY USING AIDS (EXTERNAL FORM)
- FEEL/TOUCH THE TARGETED AREA. IS IT WORKING? (INTERNAL FORM)

4. USE THE RIGHT AMOUNT OF EFFORT OR INTENSITY
- Start easily and gradually build up the effort. Work at the correct level of effort or intensity based on your health, presence of injury, experience, body age and goals
- It is OK to occasionally feel or work to a burning sensation, also called lactic acid build-up

5. AVOID OVER-LOCKING OR OVER-BENDING JOINTS
- Avoid over-straightening your joints, especially your knees and elbows
- Avoid over-bending your joints, especially your neck, knees and elbows

6. WORK AT THE RIGHT SPEED OR TEMPO WHEN EXERCISING
- Slow speed for strength and muscle building or toning and increased safety
- Faster for speed or explosive training - there is a higher risk for potential injury

7. STOP IF PAIN OCCURS
- If you feel a cold discomfort (nerve pain) or a sharp pain, joint pain or muscle strain, you need to back off the activity. When in doubt, let the area rest - there's always tomorrow.

8. RECOVERY

- If you feel dizzy, light-headed or nauseous, back off the activity. Go for a short walk for 30 seconds to 5 minutes to recover
- When you work out hard, muscle soreness can set in, usually within 24 to 48 hours later. This is called DOMS (delayed onset muscle soreness). If you experience DOMS, make sure to let your sore muscles recover. Work different body parts and stretch to recover.

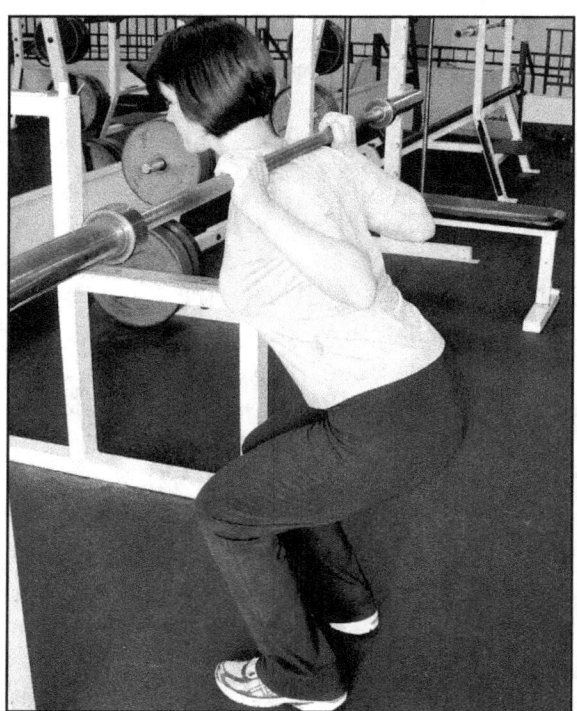

Doing a squat with correct form will ensure you get all
the benefits without hurting your knees or back.

SAMPLE WORKOUTS

SAMPLE WARM-UPS, COOL-DOWNS AND STRETCHES

In this section you'll find a few workouts you can start doing right away. At the start of each workout there is always a warm-up and stretch section and at the end there is a cool-down and stretch section.

On this page and the next you'll find simple warm-up, stretching and cool-down routines that you can use for each of the sample workouts starting on page 126.

WARM-UP AND COOL-DOWN: Do warm-ups for 3 to 10 minutes, until your body breaks into a sweat. Do cool-downs for 5 to 10 minutes at the end of your workout.

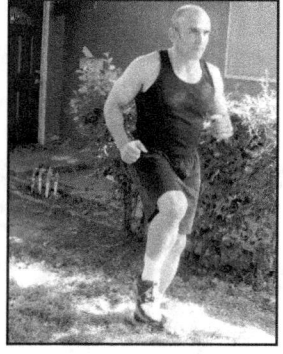

Jogging or Walking on the Spot

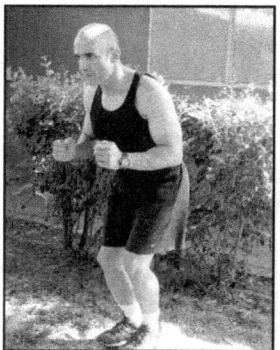

Side shuffles - 4 steps to the left, 4 to the right etc

Walk-out Burpees

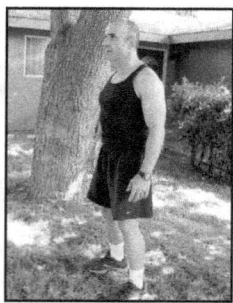 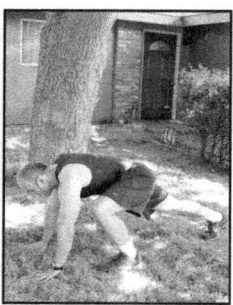 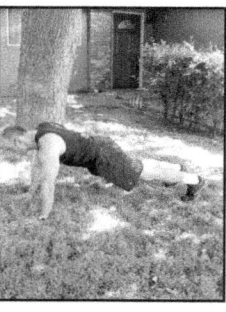 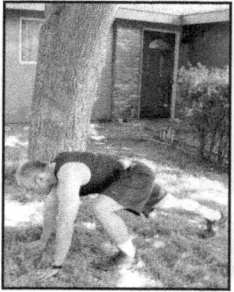 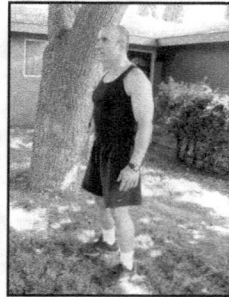

| Start position | Hands on the ground and walk feet out | Into push-up position | Walk feet back in from push-up position | Back to standing position |

STRETCHES: Do gentle movement-type stretches, move in and out of the stretches slowly. Don't bounce into a stretch.

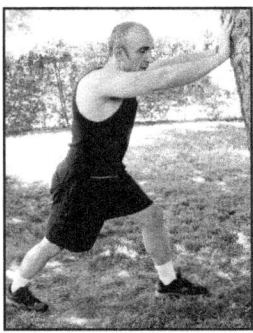

Calf stretch
(push heel down)

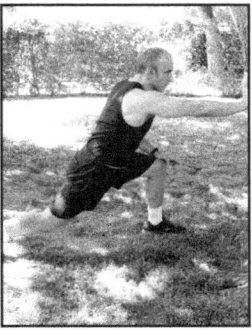

Front hip stretch
(back heel stays up)

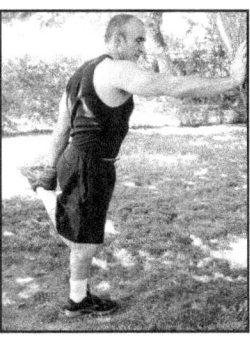

Front of thigh stretch

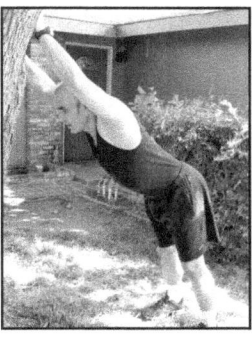

Shoulder/lats stretch

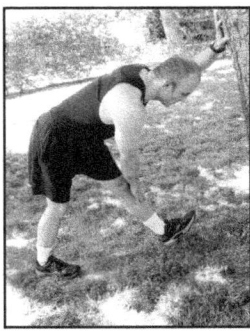

Hamstring stretch
(back of thigh, calf)

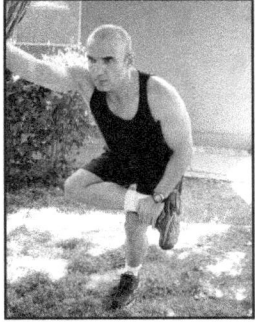

Gluteus/hip stretch
(bottom)

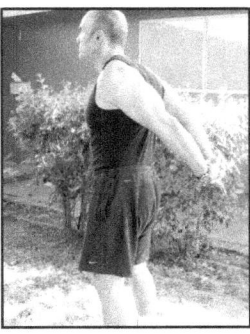

Chest and arms
stretch

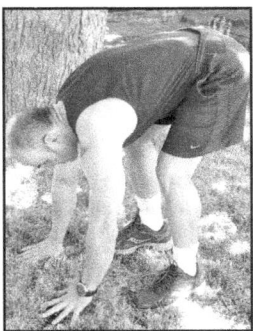

1. Touch the ground
(for lower back/
back of legs)

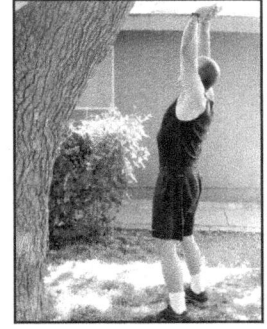

2. Reach for the sky
(for back and
shoulders)

SAMPLE BEGINNER WORKOUT

1. **WARM-UP:** Do cardio machines/calisthenics for 3 to 10 minutes until body breaks into a sweat.
2. **STRETCH:** Do gentle movement-type stretches.
3. **WORKOUT:**
   - Do each exercise for a period of 30 to 60 seconds or do 5 to 20 repetitions
   - Start with one set and gradually work up to three sets (or rounds)
   - If you have no injuries or joint problems, exercise from 50% to 70% effort, depending on your level of fitness

Exercise #1: Brisk Walk

Level 1 (Entry or Beginner fitness): Walk or skip or do a gentle jog across the floor for 30 to 60 seconds
Level 2 and 3 (Intermediate or Advanced fitness): Skip using a rope or jog for 30 to 60 seconds

Exercise #2: Push-ups

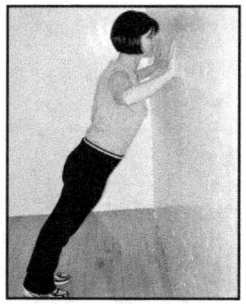

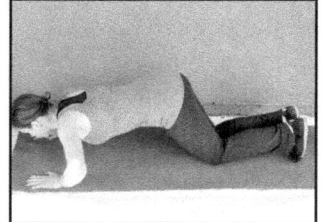

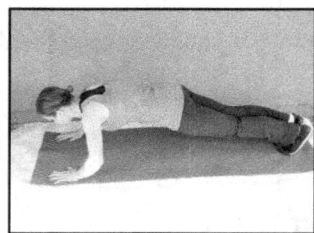

Standing Push-up

Knee Push-up

Toes Push-up

Level 1 (Entry or Beginner fitness or anyone rehabilitating a past shoulder injury and has OK to exercise): Do standing push-ups off a wall.
Level 2 and 3 (Intermediate or Advanced fitness): Do push-ups from your knees or toes. Do not let your midsection sag at any point. Keep your shoulders over your hands and lower your body until you are one inch from the ground. One breath for each repetition.

Exercise #3:   Burpees

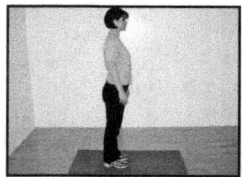 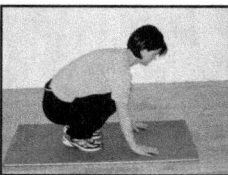 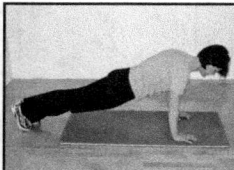 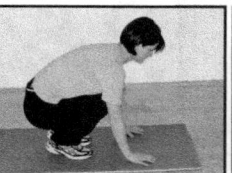 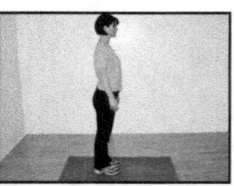

Level 1: From standing position, squat down, walk your feet back, then forward. Stand up and repeat. Do this for 30 to 60 seconds.
Level 2 and 3: From standing position, squat down and jump your feet back, then jump them forward and stand or jump up from the floor. Do this for 30 to 60 seconds.

4. **COOL-DOWN:** Do some cardio for 3 to 10 minutes; slow movements, low-impact.
5. **STRETCH:** Do gentle movement-type stretches.

SAMPLE FAT LOSS WORKOUT

1. **WARM-UP:** Do cardio machines/calisthenics for 3 to 10 minutes until body breaks into a sweat.
2. **STRETCH:** Do gentle movement-type stretches.
3. **WORKOUT:**
   - Do each exercise for a period of 30 to 60 seconds or do 5 to 20 repetitions.
   - Start with one set and gradually work up to three sets (or rounds).
   - If you have no injuries or joint problems, exercise from 70% to 90% effort, depending on your level of fitness.

Exercise #1: Burpees

Level 1: From standing position, squat down and walk your feet back, then forward. Stand up and repeat. Do this for 30 to 60 seconds.

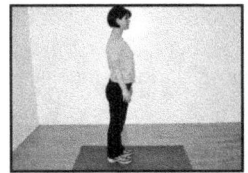 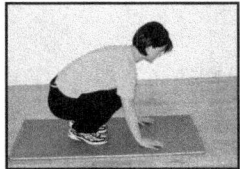 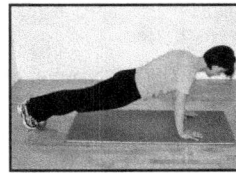 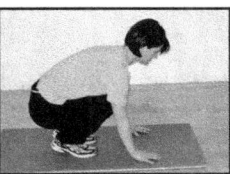 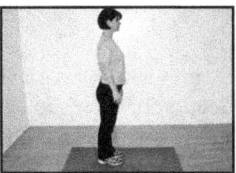

Level 2 and 3: From standing position, squat down, jump your feet back then jump them forward and stand or jump up from the floor. Do this for 30 to 60 seconds.

Exercise #2: Leg Squat to Shoulder Press

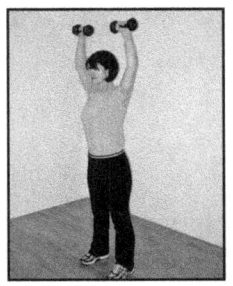 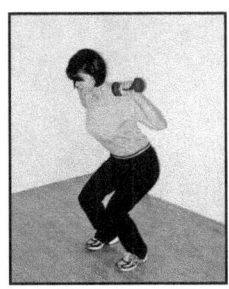 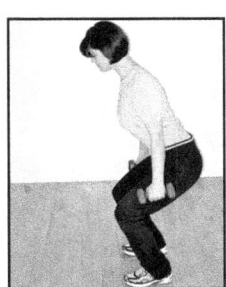 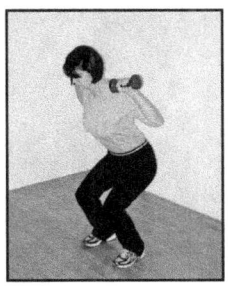 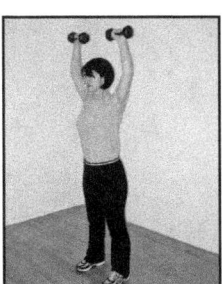

Level 1: Start with dumbbells at shoulders, lower the weight to side of thighs as you squat. Raise dumbbells to shoulders as you stand up straight. Repeat.

Level 2 and 3: Start with dumbbells raised above head, lower dumbbells to shoulders while you squat then lower dumbbells to thighs. Bring dumbbells back to shoulders and stand as you raise them above head. Repeat.

SAMPLE FAT LOSS WORKOUT

Exercise #3: Mountain Climbers

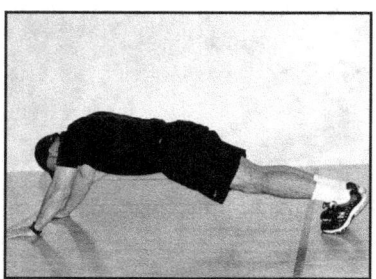 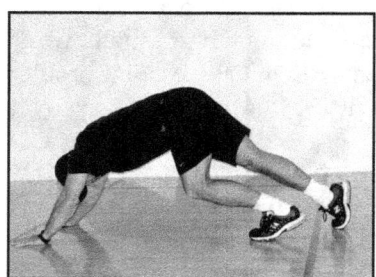

From push-up position, raise your hips, then start to shuffle your feet back and forth as if running on the spot. Keep your knees in line with your toes. Keep your back straight. Breathe.

4. **COOL-DOWN:** Do some cardio for 3 to 10 minutes; slow movements, low-impact.
5. **STRETCH:** Do gentle movement-type stretches.

SAMPLE CORE WORKOUT

1. **WARM-UP:** Do cardio machines/calisthenics for 3 to 10 minutes until body breaks into a sweat.
2. **STRETCH:** Do gentle movement-type stretches.
3. **WORKOUT:**
   - Hold each exercise for a period of 30 to 60 seconds or do 5 to 20 repetitions.
   - Start with one set and gradually work up to three sets (or rounds).
   - If you have no injuries or joint problems, exercise from 70% to 90% effort, depending on your level of fitness.

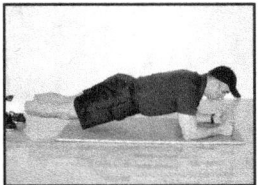

Regular Plank: Get your body into the regular push-up position, but rest on your forearms. Keep head and neck straight and arms and feet at hip width apart. Gently breathe while doing holds. Stop if you feel lower back doing the work or taking away from the abs. Do not let lower back sag. For an easier start, do the exercise with knees on the floor.

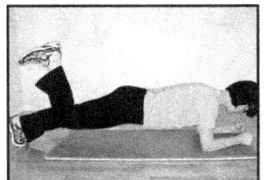

Regular Plank with One Leg Bent (Intermediate to Advanced Level): Same as for regular plank except you hold one leg bent at 90 degrees with knee off the floor for 1 to 5 seconds, then alternate to other leg. Gently breathe in and out throughout all planks.

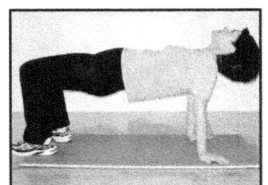

Table Top: Sit on the floor, hands by your side, feet out in front. Raise your hips and torso to the point where they are parallel to the floor. Keep your head and neck in line with your torso. Gently breathe in and out. *Avoid this exercise if you are recovering from a shoulder injury.*

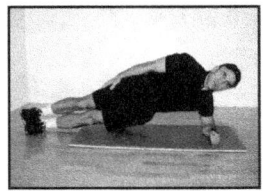

Regular Side Plank: Lie on your side, raise hips off floor and rest on your forearm and side of foot. Keep your head and body in a straight line, elbow below shoulder. Do not let your ankle over-bend; keep it straight with weight on the edge of the shoe. Resting hand can be on the floor, on the waist or held straight up in the air. *Entry Level: Bend your knees.*

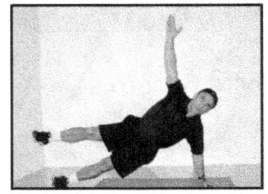

One Hand Side Plank with Leg Raise (Advanced Level Variation): Start with body weight on one hand and side of foot (keep foot straight). Have hips off the floor with one leg raised. Sequence: raise hip, then arm then leg. Hold for 1 to 5 seconds then lower in reverse order (leg, then arm, then hip). Keep head, shoulders, back and ankles in proper position.

4. **COOL-DOWN:** Do some cardio for 3 to 10 minutes; slow movements; low impact.
5. **STRETCH:** Do static/hold stretches. Stretch the whole body.

SAMPLE STRENGTH AND TONE WORKOUT

1. **WARM-UP:** Do cardio machines/calisthenics for 3 to 10 minutes until body breaks into a sweat.
2. **STRETCH:** Do gentle movement-type stretches.
3. **WORKOUT:**
   - Do not lock knee joints. Do not hold breath.
   - Do 1 to 3 sets of 5 to 20 repetitions. Use perfect form.
   - Tempo - 2 seconds down: 1 second hold: 2 seconds up. Increase to 3:2:3 then 4:3:4.

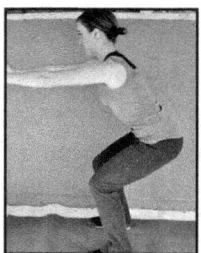
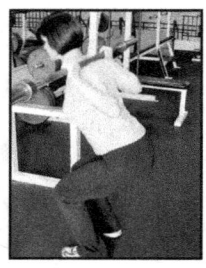

Body Squat or Barbell Squat: Feet pointed straight ahead, hip width apart. Keep natural curve in the lower back and neck. Squat until your knees are about 90 degrees. Do not lock knee joints or hold your breath.

Push-up or Bench Press: Hands slightly wider than shoulder width apart. Lower chest 1 inch off the ground (for push-up) or bring the bar 1 inch from your chest (for bench press) if you can. Do not lock elbows and make sure you breathe.

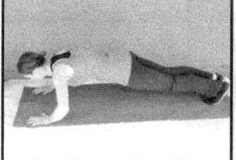
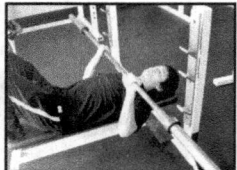

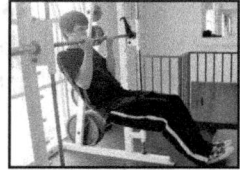
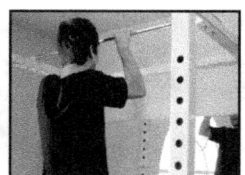

Horizontal or Vertical Chin-up: Place hands slightly wider than shoulder width apart. Pull yourself as far as you can. Keep the natural curve of the neck.

Barbell or Dumbbell Shoulder Press: Hands slightly wider than shoulder-width apart. Start 4 inches above the shoulders and press above your head. Do not lock elbows or hold your breath.

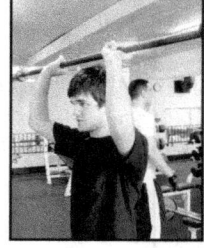
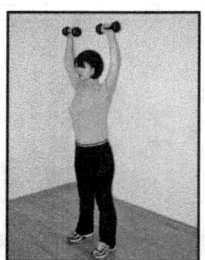

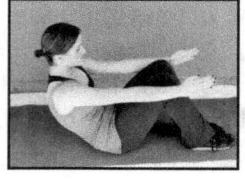
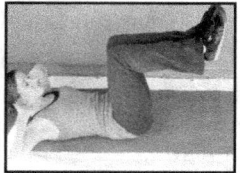

Regular Sit-up or Crunch: Keep a natural curve in your neck. With crunches, support head lightly, but don't pull on it as you crunch. Breathe.

4. **COOL-DOWN:** Do some cardio for 3 to 10 minutes; slow movements, low-impact.
5. **STRETCH:** Do static/hold stretches. Stretch the whole body.

"That some achieve great success is proof to all that others can achieve it as well."

Abraham Lincoln

LET ME KNOW HOW YOU WENT

Let Me Know How You Went

I would like to invite you to participate in the creation of the next edition of this and other books by giving your valued input on what you experienced in going through this current edition.

Please email me at rudi@gofitnow.com to let me know as directly as possible the following:

a) Your results and successes in applying the data in this book

b) What was most useful and what you liked most about this book

c) What you would like to see changed or improved in future editions

d) What other topics or information are you most be interested in learning about

SPECIAL INVITATION TO READERS TO ACCESS OUR FORTNIGHTLY FITNESS NEWSLETTER FOR FREE

Go to www.gofitnow.com to sign up for our fitness newsletter to access up-to-the-moment fitness tips, facts and more. Issues come out every two to four weeks with information coming from what successfully works for many people we train as well as current scientific studies in the fields of sports medicine, exercise science and nutrition.

ABOUT THE AUTHOR

ABOUT THE AUTHOR

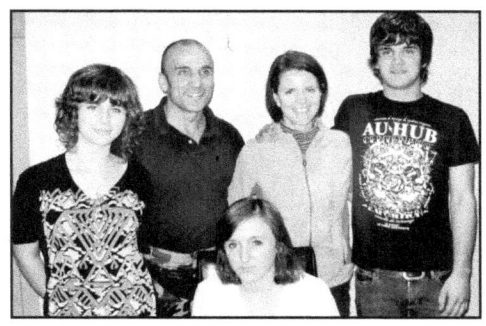

The Marashian Family. From left to right: Brie,
Rudi, Tia (front), Tracey and Obe Marashlian

Rudi Marashlian grew up in Sydney, Australia and now happily resides in sunny Los Angeles, California, with his wife, Tracey, and three children. Strongly interested in sports at a young age, it was logical to see Rudi begin a career in health and fitness in the early eighties - the "Aerobics Age", not long after playing some professional Rugby League in Sydney, Australia.

While working at VIGOR (the largest fitness chain in Australia at the time) and teaching sports to school children, Rudi studied Exercise Science at the University of New South Wales as part of the first group of fitness professionals to do so in that country.

In 1991 Rudi and Tracey purchased Mosman Gym, located in the beautiful North Shore suburb of Mosman, near Balmoral Beach and Sydney's Taronga Zoo. They successfully ran the club (well-known to locals for having good equipment and great advice with excellent service) for ten years while expanding their family to include three healthy, active children - Obe, Tia and Brie. Rudi continued delivering personal training, exercise programs, fitness testing and seminars to gym members, the public and other trainers.

In 2001 Rudi and Tracey decided a new challenge was needed and, after selling Mosman Gym, packed up the family and moved to Burbank, California. There, Rudi established a successful personal training business and decided to share his knowledge and successful actions more broadly via books and videos.

Rudi's training philosophy is, *"Real help comes when you empower through education, coaching and practice of correct and workable fitness basics. Train smart, and then train hard, using gradient steps appropriate to your level."*

www.ingramcontent.com/pod-product-compliance
Lightning Source LLC
Chambersburg PA
CBHW081829280526
45789CB00007B/2396